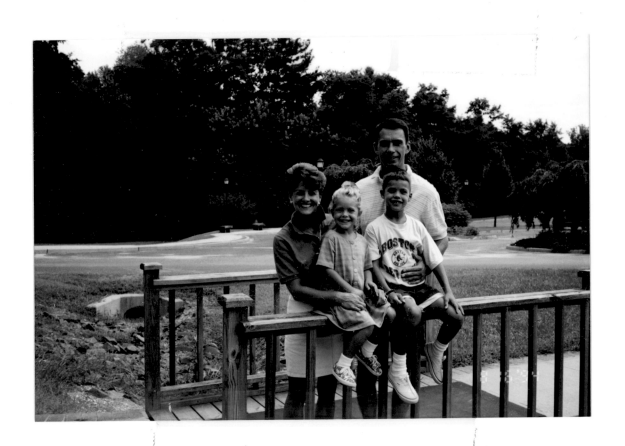

ATLAS OF

Approaches for General Surgery *of the* Dog and Cat

ATLAS OF

Approaches for General Surgery of the Dog and Cat

Mark M. Smith, VMD

Diplomate, American College of Veterinary Surgeons

Associate Professor

Don R. Waldron, DVM

Diplomate, American College of Veterinary Surgeons

Associate Professor

Department of Small Animal Clinical Sciences

Virginia-Maryland Regional College of Veterinary Medicine

Virginia Polytechnic Institute and State University

Blacksburg, Virginia

Illustrated by

Terry A. Lawrence, AMI, GNSI

W.B. SAUNDERS CO.

A Division of Harcourt Brace & Company

PHILADELPHIA   LONDON   TORONTO   MONTREAL   SYDNEY   TOKYO

W.B. SAUNDERS COMPANY
A Division of
Harcourt Brace & Company

The Curtis Center
Independence Square West
Philadelphia, Pennsylvania 19106

Library of Congress Cataloging-in-Publication Data

Smith, Mark M.

Atlas of approaches for general surgery of the dog and cat /
Mark M. Smith, Don R. Waldron.

     p.   cm.

ISBN 0–7216–3515–6

1. Dogs—Surgery—Atlases.   2. Cats—Surgery—Atlases.
   I. Waldron, Don R.   II. Title.

SF991.S597 1993

636.7′0897′0222—dc20   93-12637

Atlas of Approaches for General Surgery of the Dog and Cat   ISBN 0–7216–3515–6

Printed in the United States of America.

Last digit is the print number: 9   8   7   6   5   4   3   2   1

Foreword

If imitation is indeed the most sincere form of flattery, I must be, and am, very pleased to see this new atlas of general surgical procedures. Its format is based on *An Atlas of Surgical Approaches to the Bones and Joints of the Dog and Cat,** which has been widely used by clinicians and students in all parts of the world. There is every reason to believe that this text will prove equally appealing and useful. The illustrations are of very high quality, and the procedures described represent a high proportion of all procedures routinely performed in general small animal surgery. These procedures are well organized and written in a simple and direct style.

I perceive and anticipate an increasing need for this type of reference as our methods of teaching surgery in the veterinary colleges of North America change. These changes are driven by an increasing awareness and concern for animal welfare, not only by the public, but also by faculty and students. Far fewer dogs and cats are being used in teaching laboratories than in the past, with the increasing emphasis on simulation methodology and the use of nontraditional species such as rabbits and pigs. Although there is no longer a question of the effectiveness of these methods for teaching basic techniques, today's student has less exposure to specific operations on the living dog and cat and therefore greater need for this type of reference text. A knowledge of anatomy and basic surgical technique will allow most clinicians to perform the procedures so well described and illustrated here. The authors are to be congratulated for executing such an ambitious project so well.

---

*Piermattei DL: An Atlas of Surgical Approaches to the Bones and Joints of the Dog and Cat, 3rd ed. Philadelphia, WB Saunders, 1992.

Donald L. Piermattei
Professor of Surgery, Department of Clinical Sciences
College of Veterinary Medicine and Biomedical Sciences
Colorado State University
Fort Collins, Colorado

Preface

Surgery is visual. To feel comfortable performing surgery, one must visualize it. Review of the surgical approach and of regional anatomy is valuable prior to performing surgery to enhance recognition of anatomical structures that provide landmarks during the operative procedure. Familiarity and recognition of normal regional anatomy increases the surgeon's comfort and confidence. This comfort level is important because the disease process or tissue trauma may distort normal anatomy.

Thorough preoperative review of anatomy for general surgery currently requires the consultation of many textbooks. It is the purpose of this book to provide the veterinary surgeon with a clear, concise atlas of regional anatomy for general surgery. This textbook is written in the spirit of *An Atlas of Surgical Approaches to the Bones and Joints of the Dog and Cat* by Piermattei. Together, these books provide the veterinarian with an accessible, complete review of surgical anatomy of the dog and cat.

This book is divided into sections based on the major anatomic divisions of general surgery. Each section is composed of surgical approaches for general surgical operative procedures, often beginning with an overall review of regional anatomy relevant to the particular section. This format allows the veterinary surgeon to review specific anatomy for the operative procedure *and* to consider appropriate regional anatomy. By providing a relatively broad review, this approach best prepares the surgeon in the event that unanticipated findings necessitate a change in the intraoperative surgical plan, such as an invasive neoplastic process that requires an expanded surgical approach.

Comments made in the descriptive text reflect our experience and that of the surgeons who educated and trained us. We are grateful to our mentors and acknowledge their expertise. Overall, this book will prove helpful to all veterinarians who perform general surgery. Its review and study will miminize unnecessary surgical trauma and ultimately benefit our patients by decreasing morbidity and mortality related to surgery. It is hoped that consultation of this textbook will enable the veterinarian to *visualize* during surgery.

We are grateful for the dedicated teaching and patience of our mentors and the love and support of our families, who make possible all our professional endeavors.

Mark M. Smith
Don R. Waldron
Blacksburg, Virginia

Contents

Ear, Nose, and Throat Surgery

- Approach to the Ear Canal and Lateral Bulla

- Approach to the Lateral Aspect of the Vertical Ear Canal

- Approach to the Vertical Ear Canal

- Approach to the Medial Pinna

- Approach to the Nasal Turbinates (Dorsal): Canine

- Approach to the Nasal Turbinates (Ventral): Canine

- Approach to the Nasal Turbinates: Feline

- Approach to the Frontal Sinuses: Canine

- Approach to the Frontal Sinuses: Feline

- Approach to the Larynx (Oral)

- Approach to the Ventral Larynx (Standard)

- Approach to the Ventral Larynx (Castellated)

- Approach to the Lateral Larynx

- Approach to the Larynx

- Approach to the Nasopharynx

Approach to the Ear Canal and Lateral Bulla

INDICATIONS

Ear canal ablation and lateral bulla osteotomy for otitis externa, otitis media, and ear canal neoplasia.

DESCRIPTION OF THE PROCEDURE

A. Regional anatomy in the area of the tympanic bulla showing the facial nerve (cranial nerve VII) ventrolateral to the junction of the horizontal and vertical ear canals, and the retroarticular vein rostral to the external acoustic meatus.

B. The patient is positioned in lateral recumbency. A teardrop-shaped incision is made through skin and auricular cartilage around either the external auditory meatus or the diseased tissue occluding the meatus.

Plate 1

Approach to the Ear Canal and Lateral Bulla

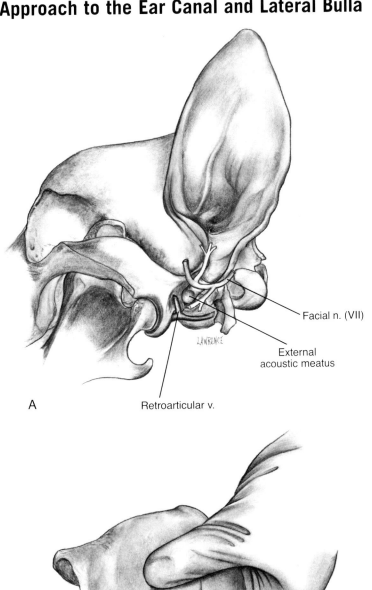

Facial n. (VII)

External
acoustic meatus

A   Retroarticular v.

Caudal

B

Approach to the Ear Canal and Lateral Bulla *continued*

DESCRIPTION OF THE PROCEDURE *continued*

C. Loose areolar tissue, fascia, and thin auricular muscular attachments are resected from the perichondrium, allowing dissection along the ear canal. The facial nerve is observed as it courses lateral and slightly ventral to the junction of the vertical and horizontal ear canals. Gentle ventral retraction of the facial nerve and parotid salivary gland protects these structures and aids in visualization of the surgical field.

D. The ear canal is transected near the external acoustic meatus. A lateral bulla osteotomy is performed by enlargement of the external acoustic meatus in a predominantly ventral direction. A curette is used to remove epithelium from the external acoustic meatus and tympanic bulla. The openings of the inner ear, located in the dorsomedial tympanic cavity and epitympanic recess, should be avoided during curettage.

CLOSURE

A soft rubber drain may be placed in the tympanic bulla and secured to skin through a secondary stab incision. Placement of sutures to decrease dead space is avoided since iatrogenic facial nerve trauma may result. Subcutaneous tissues are apposed with absorbable suture in a simple interrupted pattern followed by a T-shaped skin closure using nonabsorbable suture in a similar pattern.

COMMENTS

The ear canal is often thickened and calcified in patients with chronic otitis externa. Bone rongeurs may be required to remove the horizontal ear canal at the external acoustic meatus. Trauma to the retroarticular vein during canal removal results in marked hemorrhage. Location of this vessel in the retroarticular foramen may impede hemostasis; therefore, resection of the ear canal in this area is recommended as the last step of the surgical procedure. Packing the surgical site with sterile umbilical tape will provide hemostasis if more direct techniques fail. This material may take the place of a drain and should be removed 24 hours after surgery.

Dissection limited to the immediate perichondrial area of the ear canal will minimize the incidence of iatrogenic injury to surrounding stuctures. Trauma to the facial nerve (VII) from retraction during the operative procedure may cause paresis, which usually resolves within 30 days.

Based on a procedure of Singh GB, and Rao MM: Otitis externa in canines—its medicinal management and surgical treatment. Indian Vet J 36:236–242, 1959.

Plate 1

Approach to the Ear Canal and Lateral Bulla *continued*

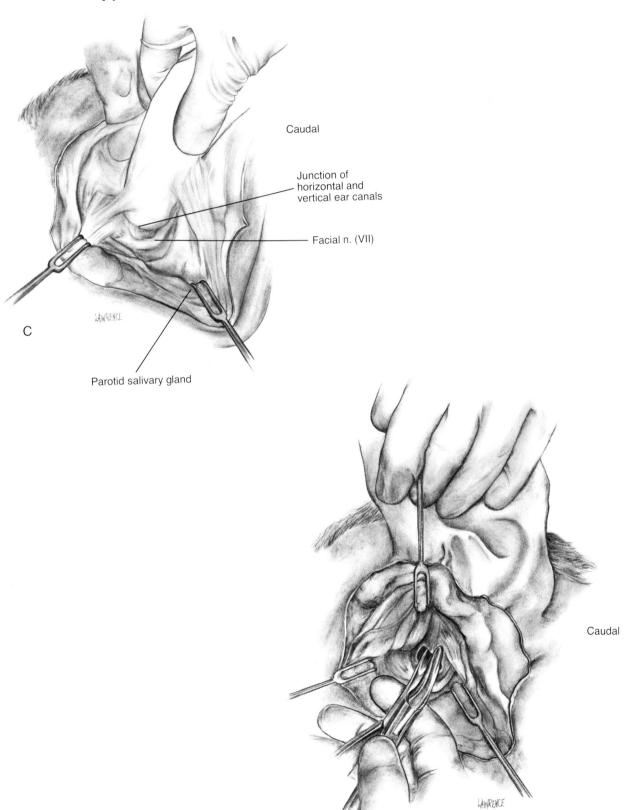

Caudal

Junction of horizontal and vertical ear canals

Facial n. (VII)

Parotid salivary gland

C

Caudal

D

Approach to the Lateral Aspect of the Vertical Ear Canal

INDICATIONS

Otitis externa and ear canal neoplasia.

DESCRIPTION OF THE PROCEDURE

A. The patient is positioned in lateral recumbency. A three-sided rectangular skin incision is made over the vertical ear canal, based at the external auditory meatus. The incision extends over the tragus cartilage and vertical ear canal ventrally to its base, dorsal to the parotid salivary gland. The width of the incision is the distance between the intertragic and tragohelicine incisures. The thin platysma muscle and subcutaneous tissues are incised, revealing subcutaneous fat, parotid salivary gland, and external auricular muscles.

B. Subcutaneous tissues and the parotidoauricularis muscle are incised to expose the vertical ear canal. The parotid salivary gland may be visualized at the ventral aspect of the vertical ear canal. The rectangular skin flap is retracted dorsally, and scissors are used to incise the vertical ear canal and the thin zygomaticoauricularis and cervicoauricularis muscles. Scissors should be directed to follow the natural course of the vertical ear canal. The cartilage incision ends at the junction of the vertical and horizontal ear canals.

Plate 2
Approach to the Lateral Aspect of the Vertical Ear Canal

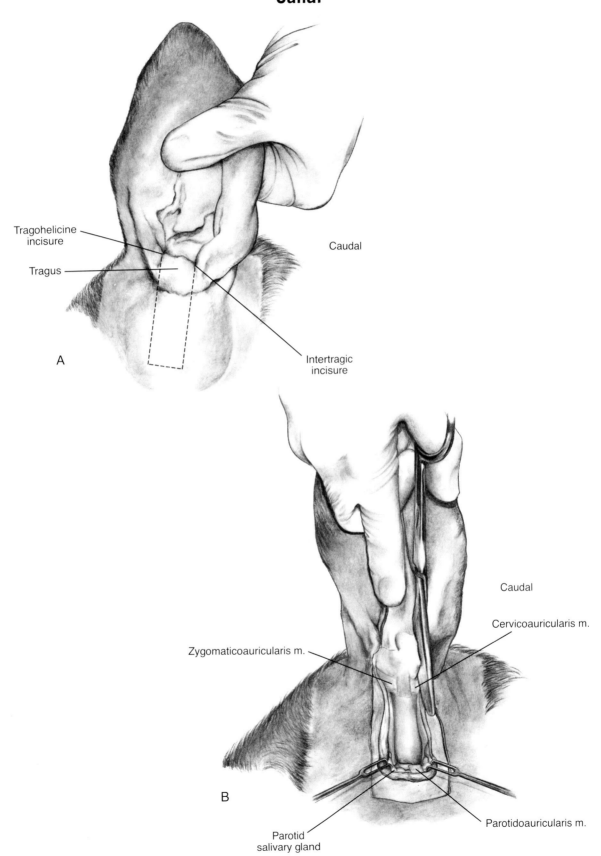

Tragohelicine incisure

Tragus

Caudal

Intertragic incisure

A

Zygomaticoauricularis m.

Cervicoauricularis m.

Caudal

B

Parotidoauricularis m.

Parotid salivary gland

Approach to the Lateral Aspect of the Vertical Ear Canal *continued*

DESCRIPTION OF THE PROCEDURE *continued*

C. The cartilage flap is reflected ventrally to ensure that the horizontal ear canal is exposed. Skin and vertical ear canal cartilage are resected, leaving a 1- to 2-cm segment of epithelialized vertical ear canal to function as a "drain board" ventral to the horizontal ear canal.

CLOSURE

Vertical ear canal epithelium and skin are apposed using nonabsorbable suture in a simple interrupted pattern. Oblique, partial-thickness placement of suture through the vertical ear canal epithelium and cartilage flap will aid closure, especially if the epithelium is friable secondary to inflammation. Initial sutures should include the four corners of the developed cartilage flap.

COMMENTS

Width of the cartilage incision should be maintained from the tragus to the horizontal canal. There is a natural tendency for the surgeon to narrow the cartilage incision as it terminates at the horizontal canal. The result is an inappropriately narrow drain board.

Trauma to the parotid salivary gland during dissection has not caused a clinical problem such as mucocele in the authors' experience.

A horizontal mattress suture of absorbable material apposing the cartilage flap and subcutaneous fascia, rather than partial incision of the cartilage, is preferred for maintenance of flap position. The latter "back-cut" may interrupt blood supply to the distal cartilage flap, causing devitalization of epithelium and cartilage.

Partial wound dehiscence, not an uncommon postoperative complication, heals readily by second intention.

Based on a procedure of Zepp CP: Surgical technique to establish drainage of the external ear canal and corrections of hematoma of the dog and cat. J Am Vet Med Assoc 115:91–92, 1949.

Plate 2

Approach to the Lateral Aspect of the Vertical Ear Canal *continued*

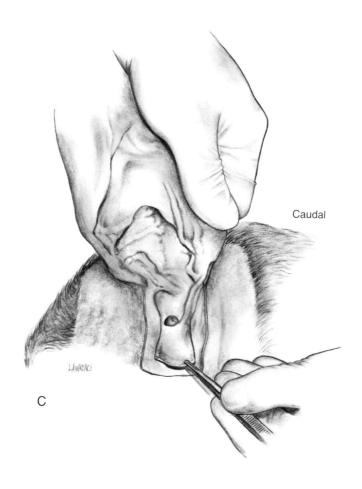

Caudal

C

Approach to the Vertical Ear Canal

INDICATIONS

Otitis externa, neoplasia, and traumatic injury limited to the vertical ear canal.

DESCRIPTION OF THE PROCEDURE

A. The patient is positioned in lateral recumbency. A teardrop-shaped incision is made through skin and auricular cartilage around either the external auditory meatus or the diseased tissue occluding the meatus.

B. Loose areolar tissue, fascia, and thin auricular muscular attachments are resected from the perichondrium, allowing dissection along the ear canal. The facial nerve is observed as it courses lateral and slightly ventral to the junction of the vertical and horizontal ear canals. Gentle ventral retraction of the facial nerve and parotid salivary gland protects these structures and aids in visualization of the surgical field.

Plate 3
Approach to the Vertical Ear Canal

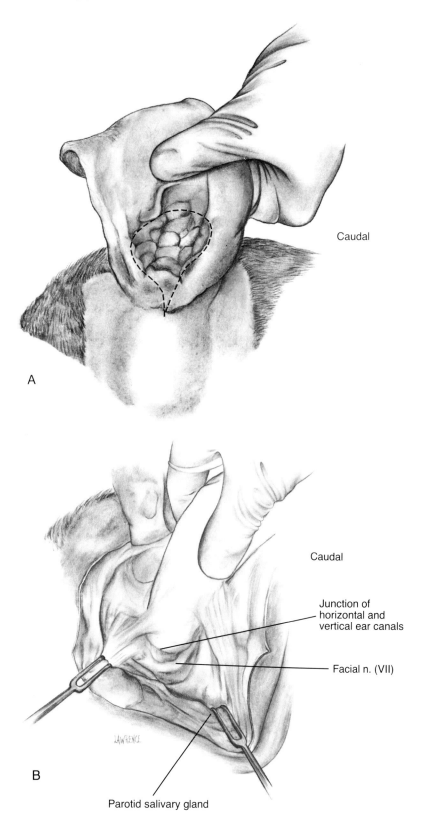

Caudal

A

Caudal

Junction of horizontal and vertical ear canals

Facial n. (VII)

Parotid salivary gland

B

Approach to the Vertical Ear Canal *continued*

DESCRIPTION OF THE PROCEDURE *continued*

C. The diseased portion of the ear canal is resected, and the distal 2 cm of the remaining canal is divided to form two cartilage flaps.

CLOSURE

The cartilage flaps are reflected ventrally and dorsally and sutured to skin using nonabsorbable suture in a simple interrupted pattern.

COMMENTS

Vertical ear canal ablation should be performed only in diseases or injuries limited to the vertical ear canal. It is unusual for disease to end abruptly at the junction of the horizontal and vertical ear canals. When there is doubt concerning the proximal extent of disease, total ear canal ablation with lateral bulla osteotomy is recommended.

Based on procedures of Siemering GH: Resection of the vertical ear canal for treatment of chronic otitis externa. J Am Anim Hosp Assoc 16:753–758, 1980; and Bojrab MJ: Modified ablation technique. In Bojrab MJ (ed): Current Techniques in Small Animal Surgery. Philadelphia, Lea & Febiger, 1981, pp 105–106.

Plate 3

Approach to the Vertical Ear Canal *continued*

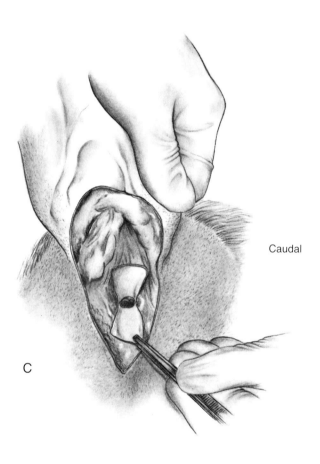

Caudal

C

Approach to the Medial Pinna

INDICATIONS

Aural hematoma.

DESCRIPTION OF THE PROCEDURE

A. An S-shaped or straight skin incision is made over the concave medial surface of the pinna. Contents of the hematoma are removed using gauze sponges and irrigation.

B. An alternative procedure provides for hematoma drainage by insertion of plastic teat cannulas at the proximal and distal aspects of the hematoma located at the medial pinna. Small stab incisions in the skin are made to place the cannulas in the hematoma. Prongs attached to the cannulas help maintain their position.

CLOSURE

Closure following standard surgical removal of the aural hematoma consists of placement of multiple mattress nonabsorbable sutures through the pinna, including medial and lateral skin and auricular cartilage. Suture placement location should be sufficient to eliminate dead space within the cartilage plates.

Cannulas are secured using nonabsorbable stay sutures through the medial pinna skin and around the hub of each cannula.

COMMENTS

Aural hematoma is usually related to head shaking as a clinical sign of otitis media or externa. The clinician should investigate the primary etiology of the disease concomitant with surgery.

Based on procedures of Ott RL: Ears. In Archibald J (ed): Canine Surgery. Santa Barbara, CA, American Veterinary Publications, 1974, pp 274–276; and Wilson JW: Treatment of aural hematoma, using a teat tube. J Am Vet Med Assoc 182:1081–1083, 1983.

Plate 4

Approach to the Medial Pinna

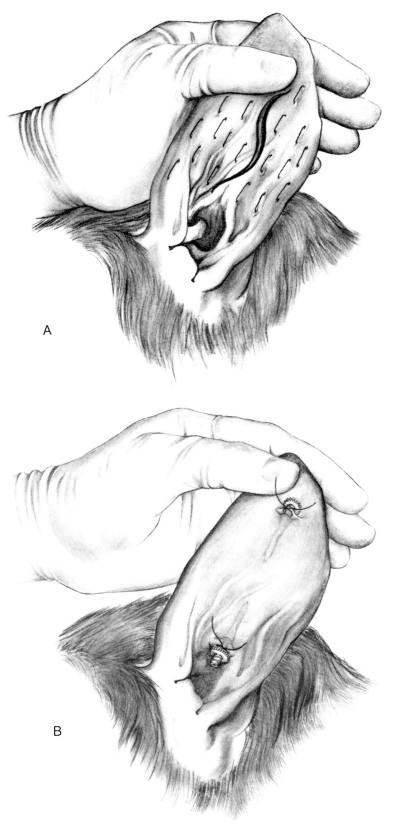

A

B

Approach to the Nasal Turbinates (Dorsal): Canine

INDICATIONS

Exploratory rhinotomy for nasal neoplasia, infection, foreign body, and incisional biopsy.

DESCRIPTION OF THE PROCEDURE

A. Lateral view of the canine skull showing regional anatomy and the relationship between the nasal cavity (dashed lines), cribriform plate, and frontal sinus. The rostral aspect of the cribriform plate is caudal to a line parallel to the infraorbital margins (ventral orbital rims).

B. Dorsal view of the canine skull showing regional anatomy and the relationship between the nasal cavity (dashed lines), cribriform plate, and frontal sinus. A line parallel to the palpable zygomatic processes of the frontal bone (dorsal orbital rims) indicates the rostral aspect of the frontal sinus. Intraoperatively, the frontomaxillary suture may be observed at the junction of the frontal sinus and nasal cavity. The cribriform plate is located medially and on midline in relation to the palpable infraorbital margins.

Plate 5
Approach to the Nasal Turbinates (Dorsal): Canine

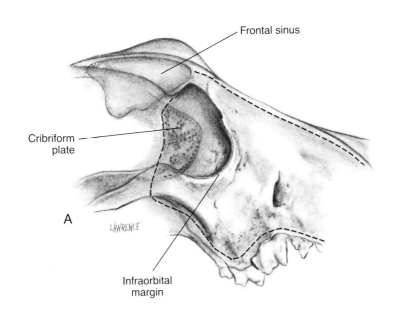

Frontal sinus

Cribriform plate

A

LAWRENCE

Infraorbital margin

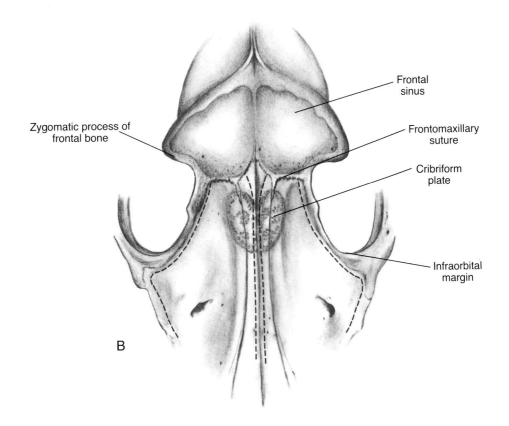

Zygomatic process of frontal bone

Frontal sinus

Frontomaxillary suture

Cribriform plate

Infraorbital margin

B

Approach to the Nasal Turbinates (Dorsal): Canine *continued*

DESCRIPTION OF THE PROCEDURE *continued*

C. The patient is positioned in ventral recumbency with the neck extended. The head is positioned over an elevated, padded area (e.g., a rolled towel) and stabilized by taping the mandible to the operating table. A dorsal midline skin incision is made beginning at the rostral end of the nasal bone and extending caudally to a location parallel to the zygomatic processes of the frontal bone.

D. Subcutaneous tissues and periosteum are incised and reflected to expose the nasal bone and nasomaxillary, frontomaxillary, and frontonasal suture lines, which represent the articulations of the nasal, frontal, and maxillary bones. Care should be taken to preserve the periosteum, which is an important tissue component of the closure. Rhinotomy is performed by using an intramedullary pin to make a nasal osteotomy on the midline, rostral to a transverse line parallel to the infraorbital margins. The planned rectangular ostectomy site (broken lines) may extend caudodorsally to the frontonasal suture line if exploration of the frontal sinus is required.

Plate 5

Approach to the Nasal Turbinates (Dorsal): Canine *continued*

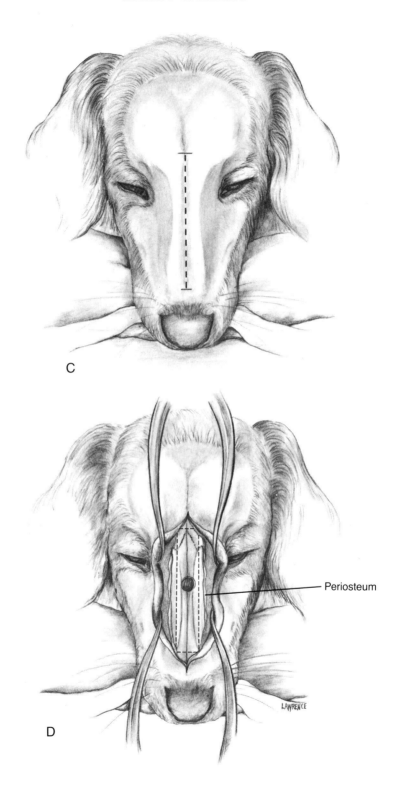

C

D

Periosteum

Approach to the Nasal Turbinates (Dorsal): Canine *continued*

DESCRIPTION OF THE PROCEDURE *continued*

E. Bone rongeurs are used to extend the circular osteotomy and expose ethmoidal conchae. In general, a narrow rectangular ostectomy is optimal, with the width determined by operative goals.

F. The frontal sinus may be visualized by caudodorsal extension of the ostectomy. The inner table of the frontal bone is removed, allowing visualization of the frontal sinus ectoturbinates and mucosa.

CLOSURE

The periosteum is apposed using synthetic absorbable suture in a simple continuous pattern. Subcutaneous tissues are apposed in a second layer, followed by skin apposition using synthetic nonabsorbable suture in a simple interrupted pattern.

COMMENTS

Ostectomy for exploratory rhinotomy may be limited to either the right or the left nasal cavity for unilateral disease.

Bone flaps may be used for rhinotomy instead of rectangular ostectomy. Fibrous and periosteal tissue healing provides firm, cosmetically satisfactory results in patients undergoing ostectomy. Infectious or neoplastic disease processes may involve the nasal and maxillary bones. Because exploratory rhinotomy is often performed to obtain tissue samples for definitive diagnosis, the authors prefer not to replace the potentially diseased bone flap.

Complete turbinectomy (either unilateral or bilateral) usually circumvents persistent hemorrhage following rhinotomy for turbinectomy. Cotton umbilical tape placed through one or both nostrils, packed in the nasal cavity, and maintained for 24 hours will provide hemostasis. A 5-Fr feeding tube placed through one nostril and into the nasopharynx for oxygen administration will help prevent postoperative complications related to hypoxia.

Based on a procedure of Spreull JSA: Surgery of the nasal cavity of the dog and cat. Vet Rec 75:105–113, 1963.

Plate 5

Approach to the Nasal Turbinates (Dorsal): Canine *continued*

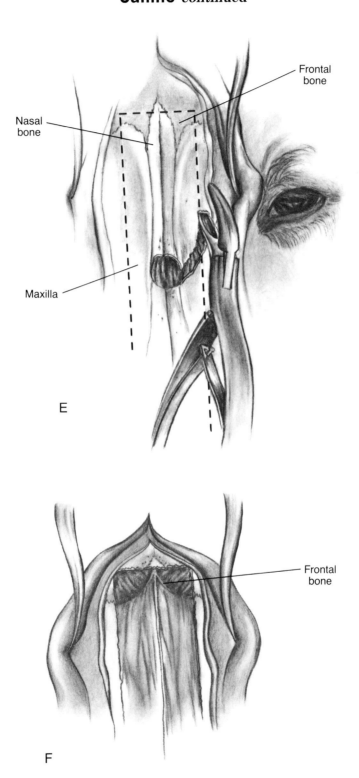

Approach to the Nasal Turbinates (Ventral): Canine

INDICATIONS

Exploratory rhinotomy for nasal neoplasia, infection, foreign body, and incisional biopsy.

DESCRIPTION OF THE PROCEDURE

A. The patient is positioned in dorsal recumbency with the neck extended. The neck is positioned over an elevated, padded area (e.g., a rolled towel) and stabilized by taping the maxilla to the operating table. The mandible is suspended to open the mouth maximally. A midline incision is made in the mucoperiosteum of the hard palate from the level of the canine teeth through the rostral third of the soft palate.

Plate 6

Approach to the Nasal Turbinates (Ventral): Canine

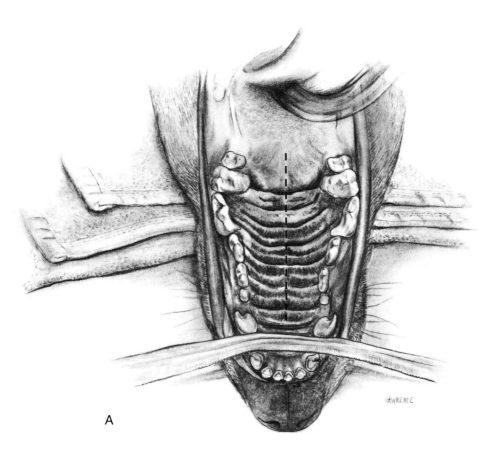

A

Approach to the Nasal Turbinates (Ventral): Canine *continued*

DESCRIPTION OF THE PROCEDURE *continued*

B. The mucoperiosteum of the hard palate is elevated bilaterally to the level of the major palatine foramen, where the major palatine artery and nerve exit the hard palate. The hard palate is removed using bone rongeurs or an air-powered drill to provide access to the basipharyngeal canal of the nasopharynx and the crest of the vomer bone.

C. Bone rongeurs are used to remove the rostral vomer bone, providing access to the endoturbinates of the caudal nasal cavity. The cribriform plate, which is located dorsally and aligned with the second maxillary molar, should be avoided. The rhinotomy may be extended laterally to the major palatine foramen and rostrally to expose additional ventral nasal meatus.

CLOSURE

The contiguous nasopharyngeal mucosa of the soft palate and submucosa of the hard palate are apposed with synthetic absorbable suture in a simple continuous pattern. The oropharyngeal mucosa of the soft palate and the hard palate mucosa are sutured with similar suture in a simple interrupted pattern.

COMMENTS

Hemostasis in the nasal cavity following the procedure may be aided by placement of gauze packing material that is brought out through the nares.

The original report of this approach recommended rhinotomy between the canine and fourth maxillary premolars. The authors have successfully applied the aforementioned modifications of the approach for operative procedures involving lesions of the caudo-ventral nasal cavity.

The ventral approach to the nasal turbinates obviates patient repositioning if carotid artery occlusion is performed to decrease nasal hemorrhage.

Based on a procedure of Holmberg DL, Fries C, Cockshutt J, et al: Ventral rhinotomy in the dog and cat. Vet Surg 18:446–449, 1989.

Plate 6

Approach to the Nasal Turbinates (Ventral): Canine *continued*

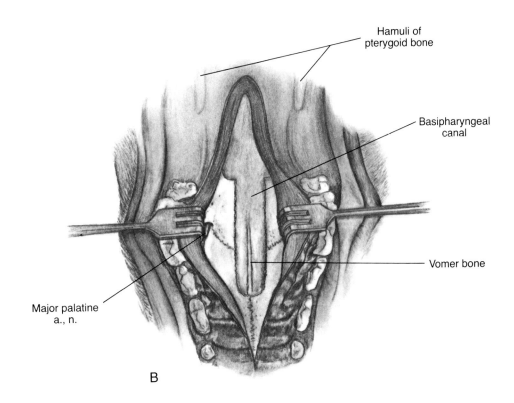

Hamuli of pterygoid bone

Basipharyngeal canal

Vomer bone

Major palatine a., n.

B

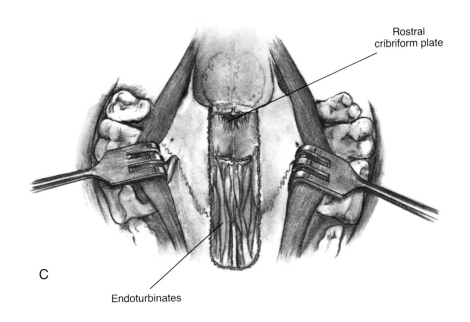

Rostral cribriform plate

C

Endoturbinates

Approach to the Nasal Turbinates: Feline

INDICATIONS

Exploratory rhinotomy for nasal neoplasia, infection, foreign body, and incisional biopsy.

DESCRIPTION OF THE PROCEDURE

A. Lateral view of the feline skull showing regional anatomy and the relationship between the nasal cavity (dashed lines), cribriform plate, and frontal sinus. The rostral aspect of the cribriform plate is on a horizontal line midway between the infraorbital margins (ventral orbital rims) and the zygomatic process of the frontal bone (dorsal orbital rims).

B. Dorsal view of the feline skull showing regional anatomy and the relationship between the nasal cavity (dashed lines), cribriform plate, and frontal sinus. A line parallel to the medial curve of the palpable zygomatic processes of the frontal bone indicates the rostral aspect of the frontal sinus. Intraoperatively, the frontonasal suture may be observed rostral to the junction of the frontal sinus and nasal cavity. The cribriform plate is located medially and on midline in relation to the palpable zygomatic processes of the frontal bone.

Plate 7
Approach to the Nasal Turbinates: Feline

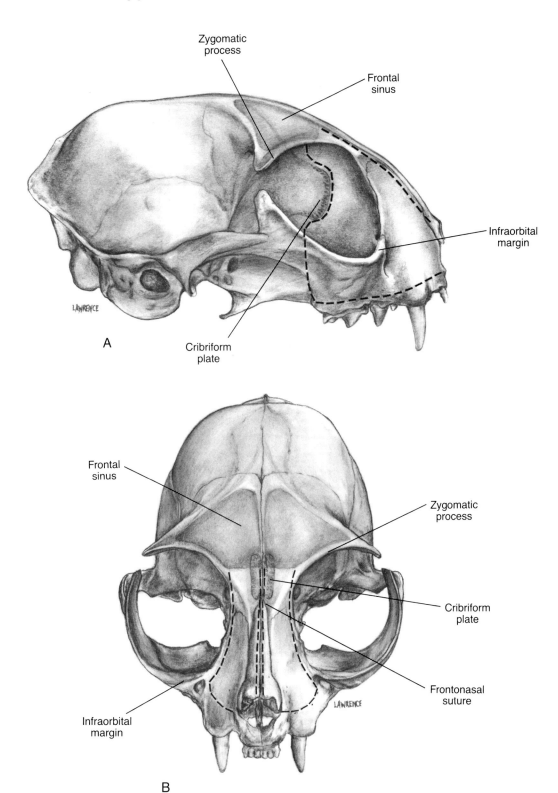

A

B

Approach to the Nasal Turbinates: Feline *continued*

DESCRIPTION OF THE PROCEDURE *continued*

C. The patient is positioned in ventral recumbency with the neck extended. The head is positioned over an elevated, padded area (e.g., a rolled towel) and stabilized by taping the mandible to the operating table. A dorsal midline skin incision is made beginning at the rostral end of the nasal bone and extending dorsocaudally to a location parallel to the zygomatic processes of the frontal bone.

D. Rhinotomy is performed for nasal cavity access and exposure of ethmoidal conchae, similar to the procedure described in Approach to the Nasal Turbinates (Dorsal): Canine (see p 16). In general, a narrow rectangular ostectomy is optimal, with the width determined by operative goals. The frontonasal suture line may be used as a landmark for caudodorsal extension of the rhinotomy. Extension of the ostectomy caudodorsally to a line parallel to the medial curve of the palpable zygomatic processes of the frontal bone allows sinusotomy for exploration of one or both frontal sinuses.

CLOSURE

The periosteum is apposed using synthetic absorbable suture in a simple continuous pattern. Subcutaneous tissues are apposed in a second layer, followed by skin apposition using synthetic nonabsorbable suture in a simple interrupted pattern.

COMMENTS

Ostectomy for exploratory rhinotomy may be limited to either the right or the left nasal cavity for unilateral disease.

The cribriform plate is well vascularized and should be avoided. Because it is not well visualized during surgery, the surgeon should be familiar with anatomic landmarks defining its location.

Bone flaps may be used for rhinotomy instead of rectangular ostectomy. Fibrous and periosteal tissue healing provides firm, cosmetically satisfactory results in patients undergoing ostectomy. Infectious or neoplastic disease processes may involve the nasal and maxillary bones. Because exploratory rhinotomy is often performed to obtain tissue samples for definitive diagnosis, the authors prefer not to replace the potentially diseased bone flap.

Based on a procedure of Spreull JSA: Surgery of the nasal cavity of the dog and cat. Vet Rec 75:105–113, 1963.

Plate 7

Approach to the Nasal Turbinates: Feline *continued*

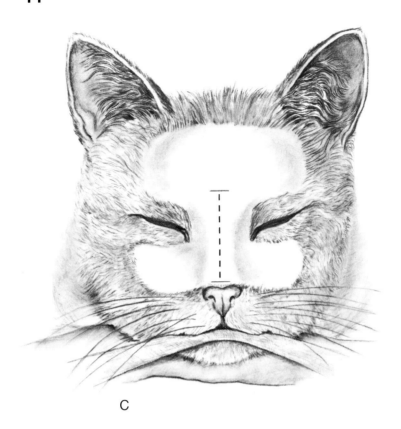

C

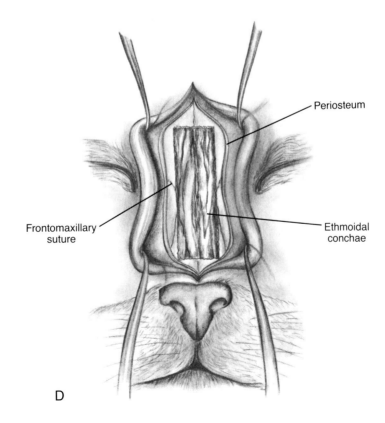

Periosteum

Frontomaxillary
suture

Ethmoidal
conchae

D

Approach to the Frontal Sinuses: Canine

INDICATIONS

Exploratory sinusotomy for neoplasia, infection, lavage and drainage, and incisional biopsy/microbial culture.

DESCRIPTION OF THE PROCEDURE

A. The patient is positioned in ventral recumbency with the neck extended. The head is positioned over an elevated, padded area (e.g., a rolled towel) and stabilized by taping the mandible to the operating table. A dorsal midline skin incision is made centered on a location that parallels the zygomatic processes of the frontal bone (dorsal orbital rims) and ends rostral to the medial canthi.

The periosteum is incised on midline and reflected using a periosteal elevator to expose paramidline frontal bone areas over the frontal sinus. An intramedullary pin may be used to perform the sinusotomy at a location that parallels the zygomatic processes of the frontal bone.

B. The sinusotomy may be enlarged using bone rongeurs to expose the caudal nasal passages for sinus drainage or to expose greater areas of the frontal sinus for sinus obliteration or reconstruction of the nasofrontal opening.

CLOSURE

The periosteum is apposed using synthetic absorbable suture in a simple continuous pattern. Subcutaneous tissues are apposed in a second layer, followed by skin apposition using synthetic nonabsorbable suture in a simple interrupted pattern.

COMMENTS

Bone flaps are not necessary. Fibrous and periosteal tissue healing provides firm, cosmetically satisfactory results in patients undergoing ostectomy for sinusotomy. A bone trephine, instead of an intramedullary pin, may be used to perform sinus osteotomy.

Normal drainage from the frontal sinus may be reestablished by placement of tubes into the frontal sinuses and through the ventromedial area of the nasofrontal opening.

Regional anatomy of the frontal sinuses may be reviewed in Approach to the Nasal Turbinates (Dorsal): Canine (see p 16).

Based on a procedure of Nelson AW, and Wykes PM: Upper respiratory system. In Slatter DH (ed): Textbook of Small Animal Surgery. Philadelphia, WB Saunders, 1985, pp 970–972.

Plate 8

Approach to the Frontal Sinuses: Canine

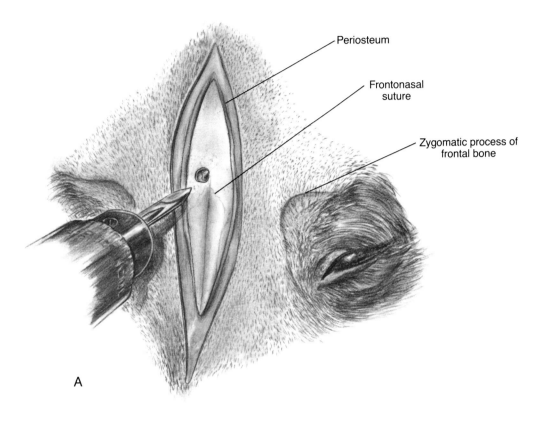

Periosteum

Frontonasal suture

Zygomatic process of frontal bone

A

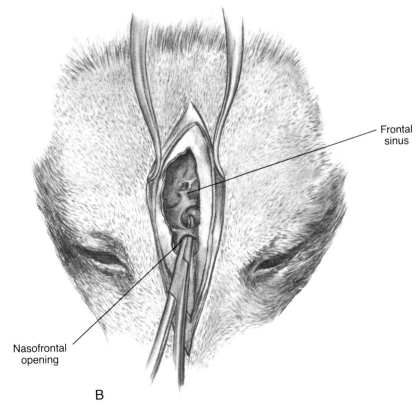

Frontal sinus

Nasofrontal opening

B

Approach to the Frontal Sinuses: Feline

INDICATIONS

Exploratory sinusotomy for neoplasia, infection, lavage and drainage, and incisional biopsy/microbial culture.

DESCRIPTION OF THE PROCEDURE

A. The patient is positioned in ventral recumbency with the neck extended. The head is positioned over an elevated, padded area (e.g., a rolled towel) and stabilized by taping the mandible to the operating table. A dorsal midline skin incision is made centered on a location that parallels the zygomatic processes of the frontal bone (dorsal orbital rims) and ending at a location that parallels the medial canthi.

B. The periosteum is incised on midline and reflected using a periosteal elevator to expose paramidline frontal bone areas over the frontal sinus. A bone trephine may be used to perform the sinusotomy rostral to a location that parallels the zygomatic processes of the frontal bone. The sinusotomy may be enlarged using bone rongeurs to expose the caudal nasal passages for sinus drainage or to expose greater areas of the frontal sinus for sinus obliteration.

CLOSURE

The periosteum is apposed using synthetic absorbable suture in a simple continuous pattern. Subcutaneous tissues are apposed in a second layer, followed by skin apposition using synthetic nonabsorbable suture in a simple interrupted pattern.

COMMENTS

Bone flaps are not necessary. Fibrous and periosteal tissue healing provides firm, cosmetically satisfactory results in patients undergoing ostectomy for sinusotomy. An intramedullary pin, instead of a bone trephine, may be used to perform sinus osteotomy.

Regional anatomy of the frontal sinuses may be reviewed in Approach to the Nasal Turbinates (Dorsal): Feline (see p 26).

Based on a procedure of Winstanley EW: Trephining frontal sinuses in the treatment of rhinitis and sinusitis in the cat. Vet Rec 95:289–292, 1974.

Plate 9
Approach to the Frontal Sinuses: Feline

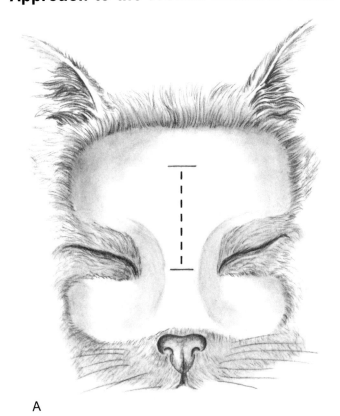

A

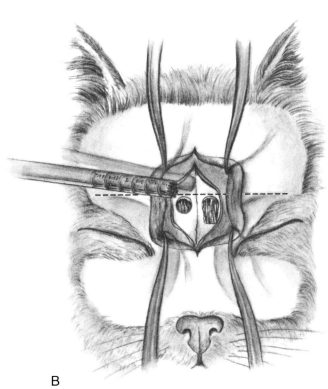

B

Approach to the Larynx (Oral)

INDICATIONS

Ventriculochordectomy and partial arytenoidectomy for treatment of laryngeal paralysis.

DESCRIPTION OF THE PROCEDURE

A. The patient is positioned in ventral recumbency with the neck extended. The neck is positioned over an elevated, padded area (e.g., a rolled towel) and stabilized by taping the mandible to the operating table. The maxilla is suspended to open the mouth maximally. The vocal folds and cartilages of the larynx are identified per os.

B. Long-handled instruments or equine uterine biopsy forceps are used to perform bilateral vocal fold resection (ventriculochordectomy) and unilateral partial resection of the corniculate process of the arytenoid cartilage. The interarytenoid groove between the arytenoid cartilages and the ventral commissure between the vocal folds are not disturbed.

CLOSURE

Laryngeal wounds are not sutured.

COMMENTS

Hemostasis is provided by intermittent tamponade of the surgical sites with a rolled gauze sponge. Suction aids visualization during surgery.

Operative wounds heal by second intention. Contraction and wound epithelialization may cause laryngeal stenosis (webbing) if either the ventral commissure or the interarytenoid groove is inadvertently included in the resection.

Although this is a relatively quick procedure, it may be associated with increased morbidity and postoperative complications when compared with other laryngoplasty techniques used for alleviation of upper airway obstruction related to laryngeal paralysis.

Per os ventriculochordectomy without partial arytenoidectomy may be performed as a debarking procedure.

Based on procedures of Anderson AC: Debarking in a kennel: technique and results. Vet Med 50:409–411, 1955; and Harvey CE, and Venker-van Haagen AJ: Surgical management of pharyngeal and laryngeal airway obstruction in the dog. Vet Clin North Am 5:515–535, 1975.

Plate 10

Approach to the Larynx (Oral)

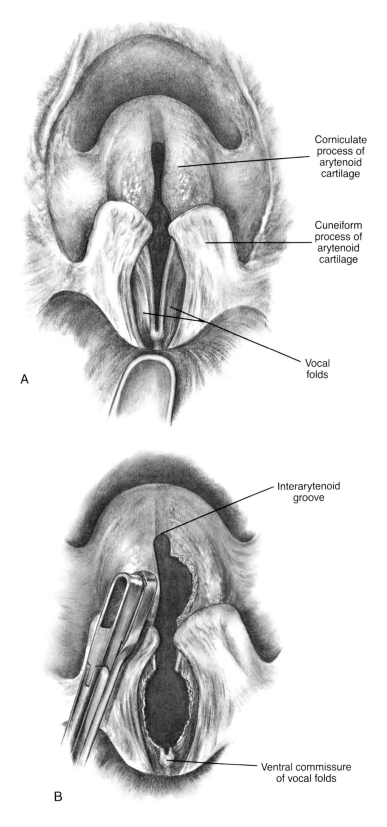

Corniculate process of arytenoid cartilage

Cuneiform process of arytenoid cartilage

Vocal folds

A

Interarytenoid groove

Ventral commissure of vocal folds

B

Approach to the Ventral Larynx (Standard)

INDICATIONS

Ventriculochordectomy, laryngeal ventriculectomy, exploratory laryngotomy for neoplasia, intraglottic stenosis, foreign body, and incisional biopsy.

DESCRIPTION OF THE PROCEDURE

A. The patient is positioned in dorsal recumbency with the neck extended. The neck is positioned over an elevated, padded area (e.g., a rolled towel) and stabilized by taping the maxilla to the operating table. A ventral midline skin incision is made over the thyroid cartilage beginning rostral to the basihyoid bone and extending caudally to the proximal tracheal area.

B. Dissecting scissors are used to incise subcutaneous tissues and divide the paired sternohyoideus muscles to expose the ventral laryngeal area. The hyoid venous arch is cranial to the laryngotomy site and should not require ligation. However, if present, the laryngeal impar vein should be ligated and divided prior to laryngotomy.

Plate 11

Approach to the Ventral Larynx (Standard)

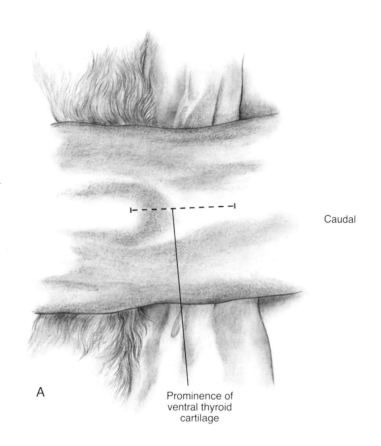

Caudal

Prominence of
ventral thyroid
cartilage

A

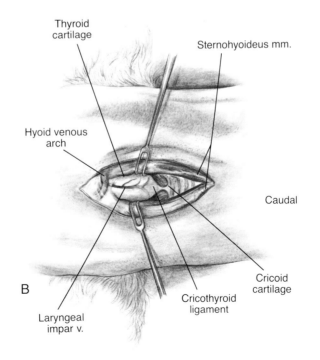

Thyroid
cartilage

Sternohyoideus mm.

Hyoid venous
arch

Caudal

Cricoid
cartilage

Cricothyroid
ligament

Laryngeal
impar v.

B

Approach to the Ventral Larynx (Standard) *continued*

DESCRIPTION OF THE PROCEDURE *continued*

C. The ventral midline laryngotomy is performed using a no. 15 scalpel blade. The cricothyroid ligament is completely incised. The thyroid cartilage is partially incised beginning caudally and extending cranially for a distance sufficient to allow visualization of the intraglottic area.

D. Ventriculochordectomy may be performed using dissecting scissors to resect the vocalis muscle from the palpable vocal process of the arytenoid cartilage and dorsocaudal attachment to the thyroid cartilage. The mucosal defect following ventriculochordectomy may be repaired by a simple continuous appositional suture (inset) using fine chromic gut or synthetic absorbable suture. Mucosal apposition may prevent intraglottic stenosis (webbing) due to healing of nonepithelialized tissue.

CLOSURE

The thyroid cartilage and cricothyroid ligament are apposed using synthetic absorbable suture in a simple interrupted pattern. The paired sternohyoideus muscles are apposed using synthetic absorbable suture in a simple interrupted pattern. Subcutaneous tissues are apposed in a third layer, followed by skin apposition using synthetic nonabsorbable suture in a simple interrupted pattern.

COMMENTS

Accidental incision of the hyoid venous arch requires the surgeon to provide hemostasis by ligation but does not cause a clinical problem.

Incision of the cricoid cartilage is not necessary for routine procedures and should be avoided.

A narrow endotracheal tube with a low-pressure cuff of sufficient size will allow manipulation of intraglottic structures. Alternatively, inhalation anesthetic may be administered by tracheostomy tube in procedures requiring extensive intraglottic manipulation. Negative sequelae related to airway compromise at the surgery site may be alleviated by maintenance of a tracheostomy tube or administration of oxygen by nasal tube.

Excision of the ventral commissure of the vocalis muscles may heal with excessive granulation tissue, leading to laryngeal stenosis (webbing). Suture closure of the laryngeal mucosa following vocal chordectomy establishes apposition of epithelialized tissue, which may prevent laryngeal stenosis.

Based on a procedure of Yoder JT: Devocalization of dogs by laryngofissure and dissection of the thyroarytenoid folds. J Am Vet Med Assoc 145:325–327, 1964.

Plate 11

Approach to the Ventral Larynx (Standard) *continued*

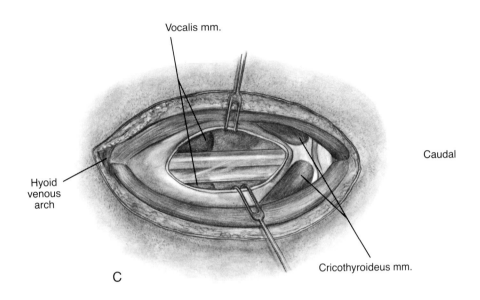

Vocalis mm.

Hyoid
venous
arch

Caudal

Cricothyroideus mm.

C

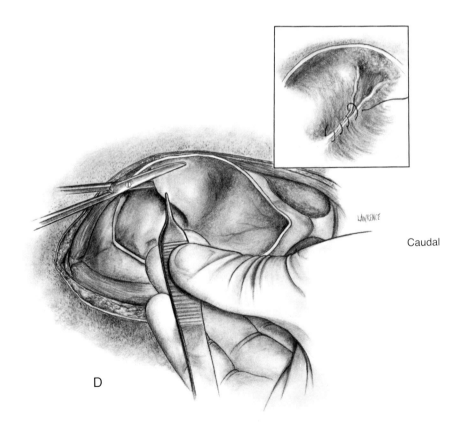

Caudal

D

Approach to the Ventral Larynx (Castellated)

INDICATIONS

Ventriculochordectomy, intraglottic arytenoid cartilage lateralization, and castellated laryngofissure as treatment for laryngeal paralysis.

DESCRIPTION OF THE PROCEDURE

A. The patient is positioned in dorsal recumbency with the neck extended. The neck is positioned over an elevated, padded area (e.g., a rolled towel) and stabilized by taping the maxilla to the operating table. A ventral midline skin incision is made over the thyroid cartilage beginning rostral to the basihyoid bone and extending caudally to the proximal tracheal area.

B. Dissecting scissors are used to incise subcutaneous tissues and divide the paired sternohyoideus muscles to expose the ventral laryngeal area. The hyoid venous arch is cranial to the laryngotomy site and should not require ligation. However, if present, the laryngeal impar vein should be ligated and divided prior to laryngotomy.

Plate 12
Approach to the Ventral Larynx (Castellated)

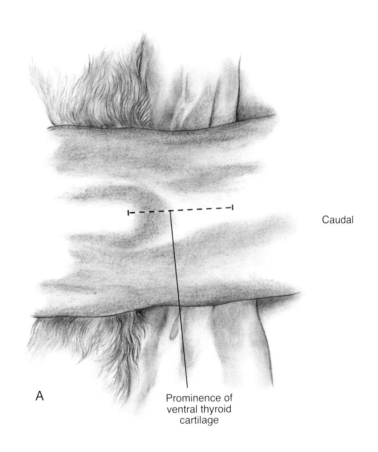

Caudal

A

Prominence of
ventral thyroid
cartilage

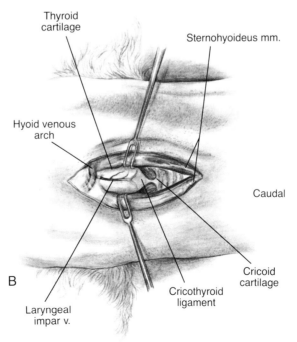

Thyroid
cartilage

Sternohyoideus mm.

Hyoid venous
arch

Caudal

B

Cricoid
cartilage

Cricothyroid
ligament

Laryngeal
impar v.

Approach to the Ventral Larynx (Castellated) *continued*

DESCRIPTION OF THE PROCEDURE *continued*

C. The ventral midline laryngotomy is performed in stepwise fashion. A no. 15 blade is used to incise flaps A, B, and C in the thyroid cartilage. Each flap is equal to one third the distance of the ventral thyroid cartilage. The incision for flap B is angled caudally, paralleling the caudal direction of the thyroid lamina. The cricothyroid ligament is completely incised to complete the laryngotomy.

D. Ventriculochordectomy may be performed using dissecting scissors to resect the vocalis muscle from the palpable vocal process of the arytenoid cartilage and dorsocaudal attachment to the thyroid cartilage. The mucosal defect following ventriculochordectomy may be repaired by a simple continuous appositional suture (inset, p 39) using fine chromic gut or synthetic absorbable suture. Mucosal apposition may prevent intraglottic stenosis (webbing) due to healing of nonepithelialized tissue.

Intraglottic arytenoid lateralization is performed by placement of a single horizontal mattress suture of nonabsorbable material through the vocal process of the arytenoid cartilage and lamina of the thyroid cartilage traversing the recess of the lateral ventricle. The suture is tied on the lateral aspect of the thyroid lamina (extraglottic).

CLOSURE

The rostral aspect of flap B is sutured around the basihyoid bone using 2-0 or 3-0 synthetic nonabsorbable suture in a simple interrupted pattern. Flaps A and B are apposed using 3-0 or 4-0 synthetic nonabsorbable suture in a simple interrupted pattern (Fig. **E**). Flap C is resected to avoid displacement into the glottic lumen. The L-shaped laryngofissure is not sutured and heals by epithelialization over granulation tissue. The paired sternohyoideus muscles are apposed using synthetic absorbable suture in a simple interrupted pattern. Subcutaneous tissues are apposed in a third layer, followed by skin apposition using synthetic nonabsorbable suture in a simple interrupted pattern.

COMMENTS

Disruption of the ventral commissure of the vocalis muscles may heal with excessive granulation tissue, leading to laryngeal stenosis (webbing). Apposition of the intralaryngeal mucosa following vocal chordectomy establishes apposition of epithelialized tissue, which may prevent laryngeal stenosis.

Inhalation anesthesia for this procedure should be administered by tracheostomy tube placed at the third and fourth tracheal rings. This tube may be removed following the patient's recovery from anesthesia.

Based on procedures of Gourley IM, Paul H, and Gregory C: Castellated laryngofissure and vocal fold resection for the treatment of laryngeal paralysis in the dog. J Am Vet Med Assoc 182:1084–1086, 1983; and Smith MM, Gourley IM, Amis TC, et al: Evaluation of a modified castellated laryngofissure for alleviation of upper airway obstruction in dogs with laryngeal paralysis. J Am Vet Med Assoc 188:1279–1283, 1986.

Plate 12
Approach to the Ventral Larynx (Castellated) *continued*

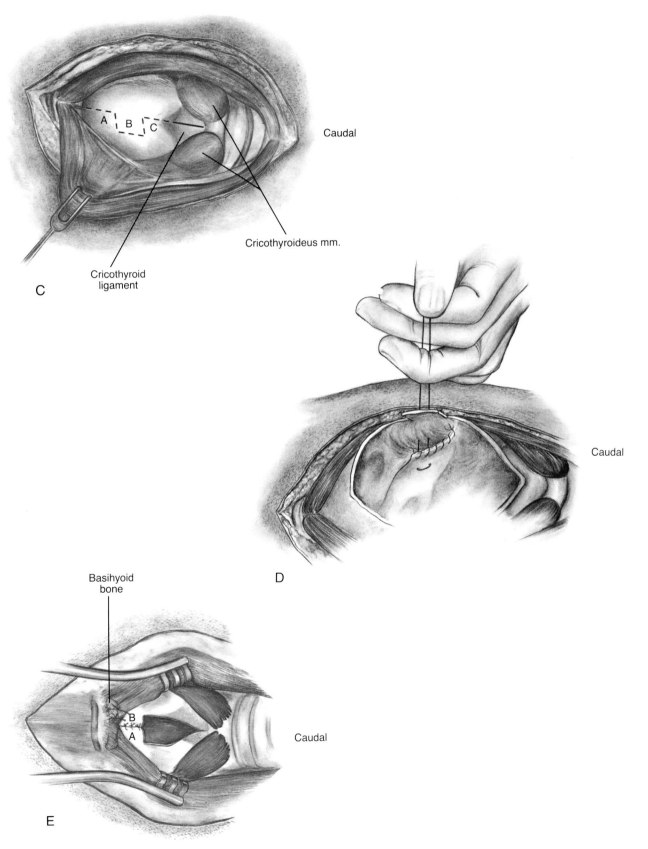

Caudal

Cricothyroideus mm.

Cricothyroid
ligament

C

Caudal

D

Basihyoid
bone

Caudal

E

Approach to the Lateral Larynx

INDICATIONS

Unilateral arytenoid cartilage lateralization for treatment of laryngeal paralysis.

DESCRIPTION OF THE PROCEDURE

A. The patient is positioned in right lateral recumbency. The neck is positioned over an elevated, padded area (e.g., a rolled towel), rotated to the right with elevation of the left mandible, and stabilized by taping the maxilla to the operating table. The incision begins at the caudal angle of the mandible and continues caudally approximately 8 cm over the dorsolateral aspect of the larynx.

B. The platysma and parotidoauricularis muscles are incised. The sternocephalicus muscle and jugular vein are retracted dorsally, and the sternohyoideus muscle is retracted ventrally to expose the laryngeal area.

Plate 13
Approach to the Lateral Larynx

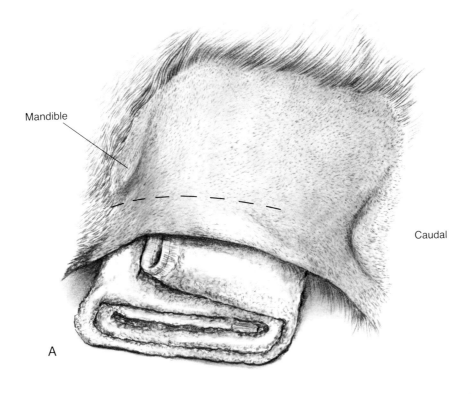

Mandible

Caudal

A

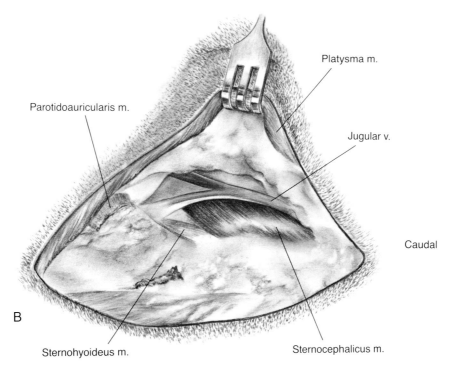

Platysma m.

Parotidoauricularis m.

Jugular v.

Caudal

B

Sternohyoideus m.

Sternocephalicus m.

Approach to the Lateral Larynx *continued*

DESCRIPTION OF THE PROCEDURE *continued*

C. A plane of dissection is established between the thyropharyngeus and sternothyroideus muscles (broken line) to the attachment of the thyropharyngeus muscle on the dorsolateral edge of the thyroid cartilage lamina.

D. The thyropharyngeus muscle is incised along its attachment to the dorsolateral edge of the thyroid cartilage lamina. A stay suture of synthetic monofilament material aids rotation and visualization of the dorsal larynx. The cricoarytenoideus dorsalis muscle is elevated from its insertion on the muscular process of the arytenoid cartilage. The cricoarytenoid articulation is disarticulated, and a synthetic, nonabsorbable, monofilament mattress suture is placed through the muscular process of the arytenoid cartilage. The procedure is continued by completion of the horizontal mattress suture over the cricoarytenoideus dorsalis muscle and through the caudodorsal midline of the cricoid cartilage. As the suture is tied, the surgical assistant observes the glottic lumen per os for adequate improvement in diameter.

CLOSURE

The thyropharyngeus muscle is apposed to its incised edge using synthetic absorbable suture material in a simple interrupted pattern. Fascial attachments of the lateral neck muscles and subcutaneous tissues are apposed using synthetic absorbable suture material in a simple interrupted pattern. Skin is apposed using synthetic nonabsorbable suture in a simple interrupted pattern.

COMMENTS

Several variations of arytenoid cartilage lateralization have been reported. The authors believe that the procedure described here successfully improves intraglottic lumen diameter in dogs with laryngeal paralysis. We do not consider incision of the dorsal interarytenoid ligament necessary to complete this procedure. However, disarticulation of the cricoarytenoid articulation allows better visualization of the muscular process of the arytenoid cartilage for suture placement, obviating multiple attempts that may fragment the muscular process and thereby jeopardize a successful result. The presence of the endotracheal tube causes lateralization of the arytenoid cartilage, requiring less tension on the lateralizing suture.

Dogs undergoing bilateral arytenoid lateralization may be predisposed to aspiration pneumonia as a postoperative complication. Aspiration pneumonia may also occur following unilateral arytenoid lateralization. Either right or left unilateral arytenoid lateralization may be performed, depending on the surgeon's preference.

Careful dissection of the thyropharyngeus muscle close to the thyroid lamina should be performed to prevent perforation of the esophagus.

Based on a procedure of Payne JT, Martin RA, and Rigg DL: Abductor muscle prosthesis for correction of laryngeal paralysis in 10 dogs and one cat. J Am Anim Hosp Assoc 26:599–604, 1990.

Plate 13
Approach to the Lateral Larynx *continued*

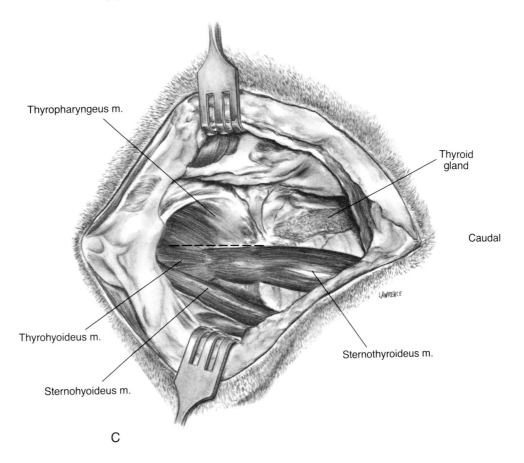

Thyropharyngeus m.

Thyroid gland

Caudal

Thyrohyoideus m.

Sternohyoideus m.

Sternothyroideus m.

LAWRENCE

C

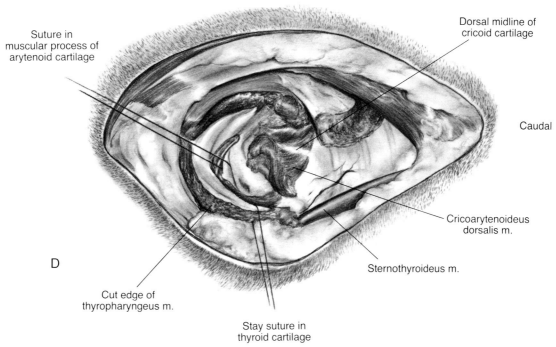

Suture in muscular process of arytenoid cartilage

Dorsal midline of cricoid cartilage

Caudal

Cricoarytenoideus dorsalis m.

Sternothyroideus m.

D

Cut edge of thyropharyngeus m.

Stay suture in thyroid cartilage

Approach to the Larynx

INDICATIONS

Laryngectomy for neoplasms of the larynx.

DESCRIPTION OF THE PROCEDURE

A. The patient is positioned in dorsal recumbency with the neck extended. The neck is positioned over an elevated, padded area (e.g., a rolled towel) and stabilized by taping the maxilla to the operating table. A ventral midline skin incision is made over the thyroid cartilage beginning rostral to the basihyoid bone and extending caudally to the proximal tracheal area.

B. Dissecting scissors are used to incise subcutaneous tissues and divide the paired sternohyoideus muscles to expose the ventral larynx and trachea. The hyoid venous arch is cranial to the laryngectomy site and is preserved if possible. However, if present, the laryngeal impar vein should be ligated and divided prior to laryngectomy.

Plate 14

Approach to the Larynx

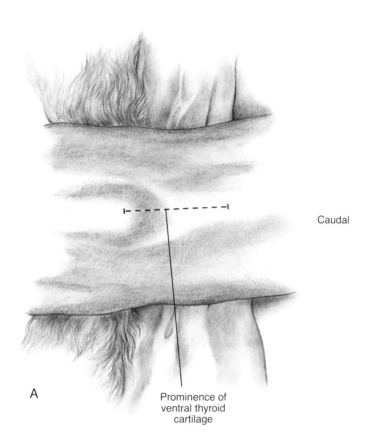

Caudal

Prominence of
ventral thyroid
cartilage

A

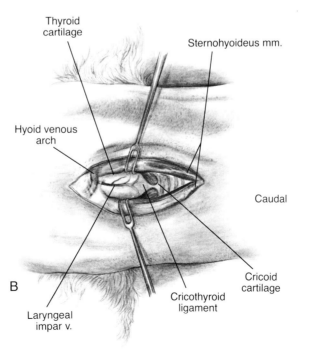

Thyroid
cartilage

Sternohyoideus mm.

Hyoid venous
arch

Caudal

Cricoid
cartilage

Cricothyroid
ligament

Laryngeal
impar v.

B

Approach to the Larynx *continued*

DESCRIPTION OF THE PROCEDURE *continued*

C. Retraction of the sternohyoideus muscles exposes the thyrohyoideus muscles coursing along the ventrolateral aspect of the larynx.

D. A bone reduction forcep is used to grasp the ventral thyroid cartilage, providing traction and lateral visualization. Dissection of the larynx is performed close to the thyroid cartilage. The thyrohyoideus muscle is resected from its insertion along the thyrohyoid bone. The cranial laryngeal artery and vein are ligated and divided. The cranial laryngeal nerve is severed. The dissection continues caudally, with resection of the thyropharyngeus and sternothyroideus muscles from their attachment on the thyroid lamina. A descending branch of the hypoglossal nerve supplies the thyrohyoideus and sternothyroideus muscles and may be severed if necessary. The thyrohyoideus and cricothyroideus muscles remain with the larynx. The dissection is performed bilaterally.

Plate 14

Approach to the Larynx *continued*

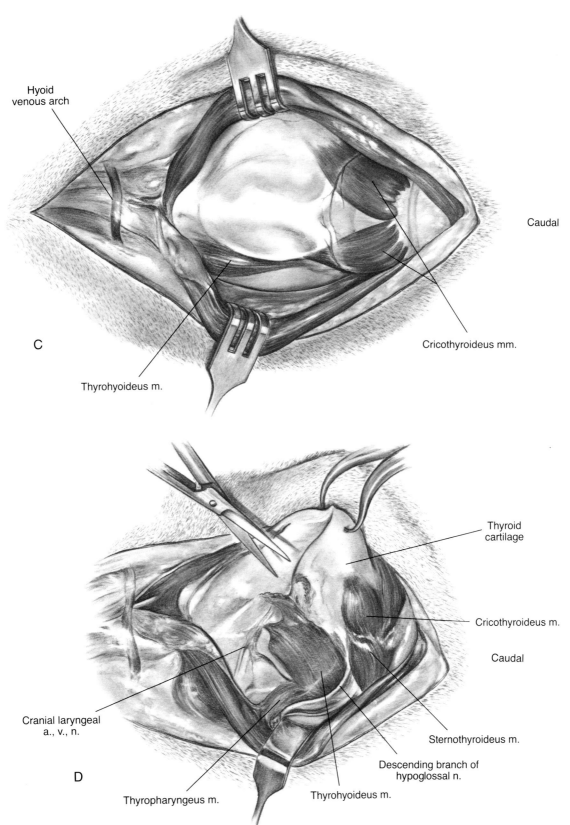

C

Hyoid venous arch

Caudal

Cricothyroideus mm.

Thyrohyoideus m.

D

Thyroid cartilage

Cricothyroideus m.

Caudal

Sternothyroideus m.

Descending branch of hypoglossal n.

Cranial laryngeal a., v., n.

Thyrohyoideus m.

Thyropharyngeus m.

Approach to the Larynx *continued*

DESCRIPTION OF THE PROCEDURE *continued*

E. Thyrohyoid bone osteotomy is performed bilaterally 1 cm caudodorsal to the articulation with the basihyoid bone. The hyoepiglotticus muscle is resected from its insertion on the ventral surface of the epiglottis. The pharyngeal mucosa is incised in a "cut and suture" manner to minimize contamination from the oropharynx. The dissection continues caudally along the dorsal aspect of the larynx and to the third tracheal ring. The caudal laryngeal nerve is cut bilaterally, and the larynx is resected between the first tracheal ring and the cricoid cartilage.

F. The first and second tracheal rings are removed, with the mucosa-lined tracheal muscle preserved to suture over the end of the trachea.

CLOSURE

The pharyngeal mucosa and tracheal stoma are closed using synthetic absorbable suture in a simple continuous pattern. A soft rubber drain is placed in the laryngeal defect and guided through a periincisional stab wound. The paired sternohyoideus muscles are apposed using synthetic absorbable suture in a simple interrupted pattern. Subcutaneous tissues are apposed in a second layer, followed by skin apposition using synthetic nonabsorbable suture in a simple interrupted pattern. The drain is secured to the skin with a simple interrupted nonabsorbable suture.

COMMENTS

Regional lymph node biopsy is recommended to stage the neoplasm.

Inhalation anesthesia must be administered through a cuffed tracheostomy tube for laryngectomy. The authors recommend that tracheostomy be performed between the eighth and ninth tracheal rings. This allows a permanent tracheostomy to be performed between the fourth and sixth tracheal rings using mucosa that has not been traumatized by tracheostomy tube placement.

Dissection performed in close contact with the larynx will minimize the possibility of iatrogenic trauma to important structures in the perilaryngeal area.

Based on a procedure of Crowe DT, Goodwin MA, and Greene CE: Total laryngectomy for laryngeal mast cell tumor in a dog. J Am Anim Hosp Assoc 22:809–816, 1986.

Plate 14

Approach to the Larynx *continued*

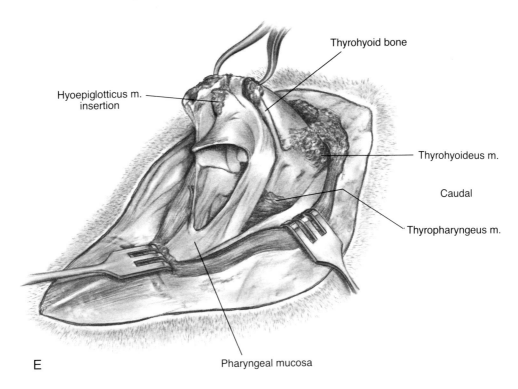

Hyoepiglotticus m. insertion

Thyrohyoid bone

Thyrohyoideus m.

Caudal

Thyropharyngeus m.

Pharyngeal mucosa

E

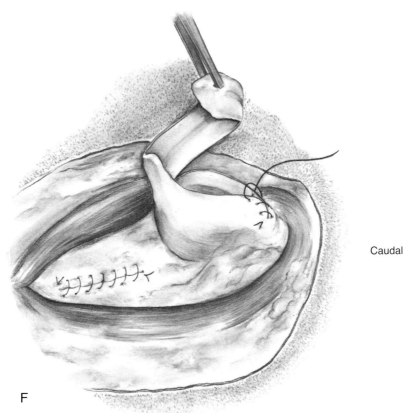

Caudal

F

Approach to the Nasopharynx

INDICATIONS

Exploratory surgery for nasopharyngeal polyp, neoplasm, and foreign body.

DESCRIPTION OF THE PROCEDURE

A. The patient is positioned in dorsal recumbency with the neck extended. The neck is positioned over an elevated, padded area (e.g., a rolled towel) and stabilized by taping the maxilla to the operating table. The mandible is suspended to open the mouth maximally.

B. Stay sutures are placed in each side of the caudal soft palate to provide traction. A ventral midline incision is made through the oropharyngeal mucosa, the palatinus muscle, and the nasopharyngeal mucosa.

CLOSURE

The nasopharyngeal mucosa is apposed in a caudal to rostral direction using synthetic absorbable suture in a simple continuous pattern. The palatinus muscle and oropharyngeal mucosa are apposed using similar suture in a simple interrupted pattern.

COMMENTS

Rostral displacement of the soft palate by traction with a blunt hooked instrument will often provide adequate visualization for nasopharyngeal surgery, making soft palate incision unnecessary.

Based on a procedure of Nelson AW, and Wykes PM: Upper respiratory system. In *Slatter DH (ed): Textbook of Small Animal Surgery. Philadelphia, WB Saunders, 1985, p 968.*

Plate 15

Approach to the Nasopharynx

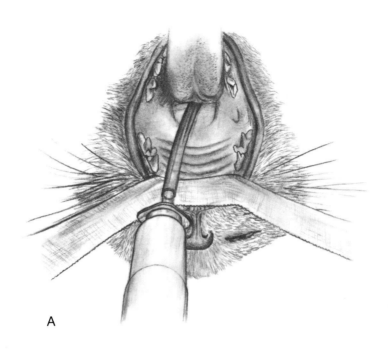

A

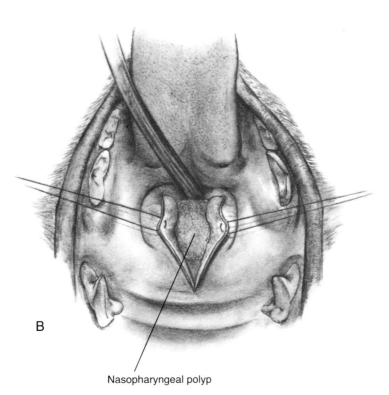

B

Nasopharyngeal polyp

Oral and Maxillofacial Surgery

Approach to the Lateral Premaxilla

INDICATIONS

Resective surgery for neoplasia or limited premaxillectomy for oronasal fistula.

DESCRIPTION OF THE PROCEDURE

A. The patient is positioned in lateral recumbency. The buccal mucosa is incised at least 1 cm from the lesion. A periosteal elevator is used to elevate the mucosa from its attachment on the maxilla and incisive bones. The infraorbital artery, vein, and nerve exit the infraorbital canal of the maxilla and should be avoided unless wide resection requires their division and ligation.

B. The palatal mucosa is incised similarly, and the mucoperiosteum is elevated. The major palatine artery is divided and ligated if the resection approaches the major palatine foramen.

C. Resection of the premaxilla and/or maxilla exposes the nasal cavity.

CLOSURE

The buccal mucosa is undermined to allow tension-free apposition to palatal mucosa. A two-layer closure is performed using synthetic absorbable suture in simple interrupted patterns for the submucosa and mucosa.

COMMENTS

Maxillectomy may be performed with an oscillating bone saw or osteotome and mallet after scoring the osteotomy lines with small perforating holes.

Nasal turbinectomy should be performed if the neoplasm invades the nasal cavity.

Premaxillectomy and partial maxillectomy are limited by the surgeon's ability to reconstruct the oronasal defect. Patients with lesions that cross midline are usually not considered candidates for partial maxillectomy. Tension-free closure is imperative to prevent wound dehiscence and subsequent oronasal fistula. Failure of second-intention healing for partial wound dehiscence requires utilization of oronasal fistula repair techniques.

Food should be liquid in consistency during the first postoperative week.

Cosmesis is generally good following surgery. Observable surgical results, including facial concavity and an elevated lip, do not affect function and are usually accepted by the owner.

Based on procedures of Withrow SJ, Nelson AW, Manley PA, et al: Premaxillectomy in the dog. J Am Anim Hosp Assoc 21:49–55, 1985; and Salisbury SK, Thackee HL, Pantzer EE, et al: Partial maxillectomy in the dog: comparison of suture materials and closure techniques. Vet Surg 14:265–276, 1985.

Plate 16

Approach to the Lateral Premaxilla

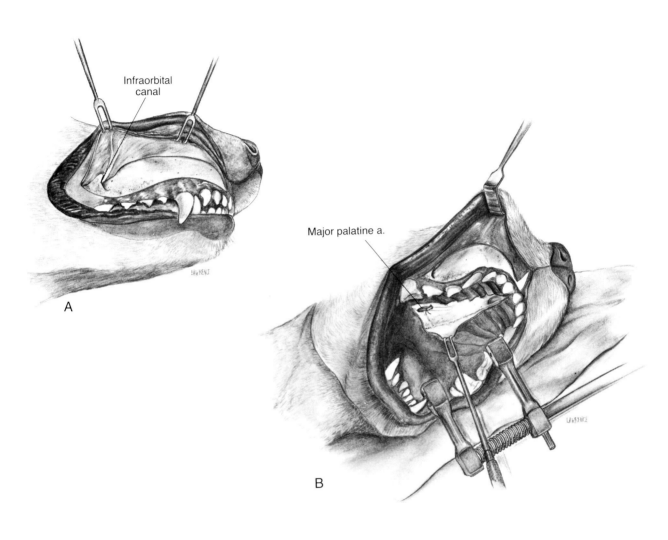

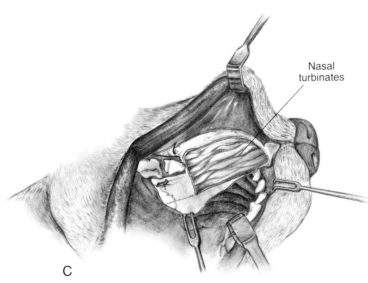

Approach to the Lateral Maxilla: Feline

INDICATIONS

Resective surgery for neoplasia or limited premaxillectomy for oronasal fistula.

DESCRIPTION OF THE PROCEDURE

A. The patient is positioned in lateral recumbency. The buccal mucosa is incised at least 1 cm from the lesion. A periosteal elevator is used to elevate the mucosa from its attachment on the maxilla and incisive bones. The palatal mucosa is incised similarly, and the mucoperiosteum is elevated. The major palatine artery is divided and ligated if the resection approaches the major palatine foramen.

B. The infraorbital artery, vein, and nerve exiting the infraorbital canal of the maxilla are divided. Further subperiosteal elevation is performed to free soft tissue attachments from the dorsal maxilla, exposing the dorsal nasal vein and the origin of the masseter muscle on the ventral zygomatic arch.

C. Resection of the lateral maxilla, incisive, and palatine bones exposes the nasal cavity.

CLOSURE

The buccal mucosa is undermined to allow tension-free apposition to palatal mucosa. A two-layer closure is performed using synthetic absorbable suture in simple interrupted patterns for the submucosa and mucosa.

COMMENTS

Maxillectomy may be performed with an oscillating bone saw or osteotome and mallet after scoring the osteotomy lines with small perforating holes.

Nasal turbinectomy should be performed if the neoplasm invades the nasal cavity.

Maxillectomy is limited by the surgeon's ability to reconstruct the oronasal defect. Patients with lesions that cross midline are usually not considered candidates for maxillectomy. Tension-free closure is imperative to prevent wound dehiscence and subsequent oronasal fistula. If wound dehiscence occurs, second-intention healing is usually successful. Failure of second-intention healing requires utilization of oronasal fistula repair techniques.

Food should be liquid in consistency during the first postoperative week.

Cosmesis is generally good following surgery. Observable surgical results, including facial concavity and an elevated lip, do not affect function and are usually accepted by the owner.

Based on a procedure of Salisbury SK, Richardson DC, and Lantz GC: Partial maxillectomy and premaxillectomy in the treatment of oral neoplasia in the dog and cat. Vet Surg 15:16–26, 1986.

Plate 17
Approach to the Lateral Maxilla: Feline

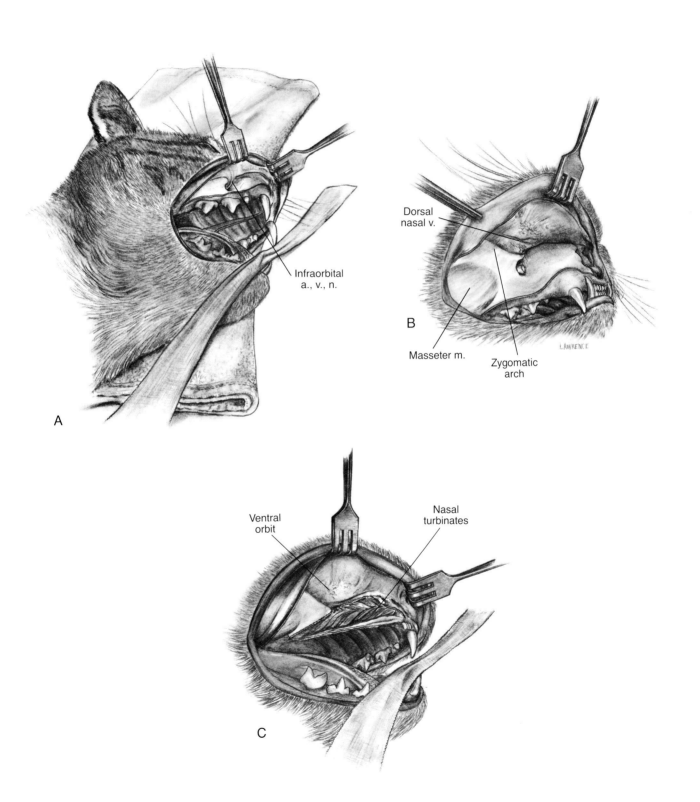

A

Infraorbital
a., v., n.

B

Dorsal
nasal v.

Masseter m.

Zygomatic
arch

LAWRENCE

C

Ventral
orbit

Nasal
turbinates

Approach to the Lateral Maxilla: Canine

INDICATIONS

Resective surgery for neoplasia.

DESCRIPTION OF THE PROCEDURE

A. The patient is positioned in lateral recumbency. The buccal mucosa is incised at least 1 cm from the lesion. A periosteal elevator is used to elevate the mucosa from its attachment on the maxilla and incisive bones. The infraorbital artery, vein, and nerve are divided as they exit the infraorbital canal of the maxilla. The facial vein requires division and ligation near the levator nasolabialis muscle and as it joins the deep facial vein. The zygomatic bone is exposed by elevation of periosteum and sharp incision of the insertion of the masseter muscle. The palatal mucosa is incised at least 1 cm from the lesion, and the mucoperiosteum is elevated. The incision is continued caudally through the lateral soft palate to join the incised buccal mucosa. The major palatine artery is divided and ligated if the resection approaches the major palatine foramen.

Plate 18
Approach to the Lateral Maxilla: Canine

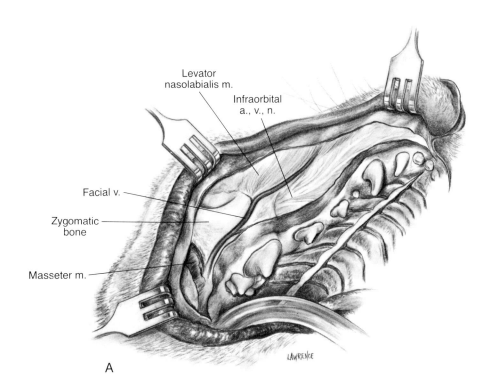

Levator nasolabialis m.

Infraorbital a., v., n.

Facial v.

Zygomatic bone

Masseter m.

LAWRENCE

A

Approach to the Lateral Maxilla: Canine *continued*

DESCRIPTION OF THE PROCEDURE *continued*

B. A blunt instrument is placed on the medial aspect of the zygomatic bone to protect orbital contents during zygomatic osteotomy. Resection of the lateral maxilla, incisive, and palatine bones exposes the nasal cavity. Arterial hemorrhage is encountered from the more proximal aspect of the infraorbital artery as the infraorbital canal is disrupted. The deep facial vein is observed near the periorbital fat and zygomatic salivary gland.

CLOSURE

The buccal mucosa is undermined to allow tension-free apposition to palatal mucosa. A two-layer closure is performed using synthetic absorbable suture in simple interrupted patterns for the submucosa and mucosa.

COMMENTS

Maxillectomy may be performed with an oscillating bone saw or osteotome and mallet after scoring the osteotomy lines with small perforating holes.

Nasal turbinectomy should be performed if the neoplasm invades the nasal cavity.

Maxillectomy is limited by the surgeon's ability to reconstruct the oronasal defect. Patients with lesions that cross midline are usually not considered candidates for partial maxillectomy. Tension-free closure is imperative to prevent wound dehiscence and subsequent oronasal fistula. If wound dehiscence occurs, second-intention healing is usually successful. Failure of second-intention healing requires utilization of oronasal fistula repair techniques.

Full-thickness incision of the lip commissure, which may be performed to gain exposure of the caudal operative field, requires closure of oral mucosa, muscle, and skin in individual layers.

Food should be liquid in consistency during the first postoperative week.

Cosmesis is generally good following surgery. Observable surgical results, including facial concavity and an elevated lip, do not affect function and are usually accepted by the owner.

Based on a procedure of Salisbury SK, Richardson DC, and Lantz GC: Partial maxillectomy and premaxillectomy in the treatment of oral neoplasia in the dog and cat. Vet Surg 15:16–26, 1986.

Plate 18

Approach to the Lateral Maxilla: Canine *continued*

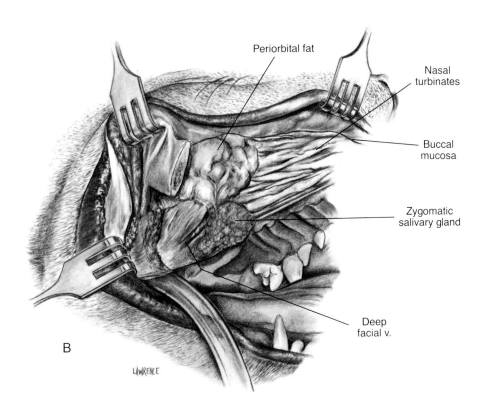

Periorbital fat

Nasal turbinates

Buccal mucosa

Zygomatic salivary gland

Deep facial v.

B

LAWRENCE

Approach to the Rostral Maxilla

INDICATIONS

Resective surgery for neoplasia.

DESCRIPTION OF THE PROCEDURE

A. The patient is positioned in dorsal recumbency. The lateral and rostral buccal mucosae and hard palate mucoperiosteum are incised at least 1 cm from the lesion. A periosteal elevator is used to elevate mucosa from its attachment on the hard palate, maxilla, and incisive bones.

B. The cartilaginous nasal fossae and septum are incised, and soft tissues are elevated caudally to the osteotomy site. Rostral maxillectomy is performed using an oscillating bone saw or osteotome and mallet after scoring the osteotomy lines with small perforating holes. Maxilloturbinates are transected along the plane of maxillectomy. Hemorrhage is controlled by electrocautery, direct pressure, and vessel ligation.

CLOSURE

The premaxillary defect may be reconstructed using buccal mucosal flaps to provide nasal and oral mucosal surfaces. The two-layer closure is performed using synthetic absorbable suture in simple interrupted patterns. Alternatively, the buccal mucosa may be apposed to hard palate mucoperiosteum in a primary two-layer closure using synthetic absorbable suture in simple interrupted patterns for the submucosa and mucosa.

COMMENTS

Rostral maxillectomy caudal to the level of the maxillary first premolar results in shortening of the nose.

Wound dehiscence is uncommon and heals by second intention or requires a second, minor revision surgery.

Food should be liquid in consistency during the first postoperative week.

Whether the nasolacrimal duct is transected or ligated, the patient may have an intermittent serous discharge resulting in crusting of the nares and epiphora. The authors make no effort to ligate the nasolacrimal duct.

Cosmesis is generally good following surgery. Observable surgical results, including drooping of the nose ventrally and displacement of the maxillary lip caudal to the mandibular canine teeth, do not affect function and are usually accepted by the owner.

Based on procedures of Withrow SJ, Nelson AW, Manley PA, et al: Premaxillectomy in the dog. J Am Anim Hosp Assoc 21:49–55, 1985; and Salisbury SK, Thackee HL, Pantzer EE, et al: Partial maxillectomy in the dog: comparison of suture materials and closure techniques. Vet Surg 14:265–276, 1985.

Plate 19

Approach to the Rostral Maxilla

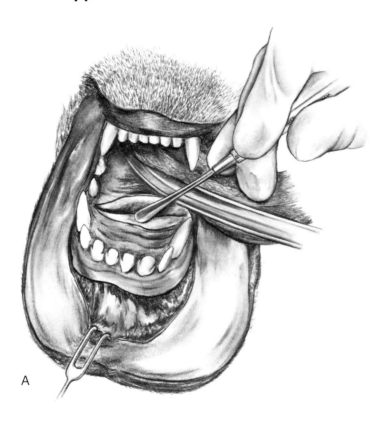

A

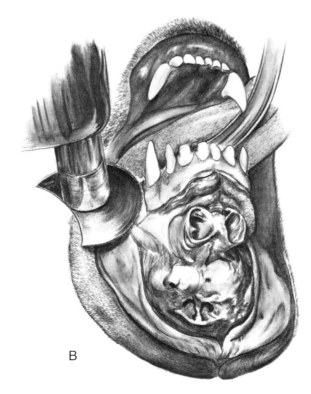

B

Approach to the Rostral Mandible: Feline

INDICATIONS

Unilateral or bilateral mandibulectomy for neoplasms of the rostral mandible, nonunion, and chronic osteomyelitis.

DESCRIPTION OF THE PROCEDURE

A. The patient is positioned in dorsal recumbency. The patient's neck is extended over an elevated, padded area (e.g., a rolled towel), and the maxilla is secured to the operating table using adhesive tape. Thumb forceps are used to retract skin of the ventral mandible to expose oral mucosa. The oral and labial mucosae should be incised a minimum of 1 cm from the periphery of the neoplasm.

B. Sharp dissection is performed using scalpel or periosteal elevator to incise soft tissues, including the oral mucosa, and the mentalis, orbicularis oris, mylohyoideus, and geniohyoideus muscles from the rostral mandible. Dissection extends to the level of mandibulectomy.

C. Mandibulectomy is usually performed rostral to the frenulum of the tongue at the level of the mandibular third premolar. Ostectomy sites are contoured with bone rongeurs to facilitate closure and remove sharp bone edges that may traumatize mucosa.

CLOSURE

The wound is closed in one layer, because the oral mucosa is thin. The oral and labial mucosae are apposed in a simple continuous or interrupted pattern using synthetic or natural absorbable suture. Provision for ventral drainage is usually not necessary.

COMMENTS

A pharyngostomy for endotracheal tube placement facilitates extensive oral surgery.

Bone wax is a foreign substance that may disrupt wound healing. Its application is not necessary for hemostasis at mandibulectomy sites. Mandibular body stabilization following resection is not necessary.

Full-thickness lip excision may be required to restore acceptable cosmesis. Resection of a triangular shape with its base along the mucocutaneous junction shortens the lip, which must be sutured to oral mucosa.

Wound dehiscence over the resected mandible may occur and resolves by second-intention healing with conservative management.

Food should be liquid in consistency during the first postoperative week.

Tongue protrusion may occur following surgery; however, patients usually adapt to maintain the tongue retracted into the oral cavity. Cheiloplasty may be required to shorten the lip commissure to prevent tongue protrusion. In the authors' experience, owners rarely complain about cosmesis following this procedure.

Based on procedures of Vernon FF, and Helphrey M: Rostral mandibulectomy: three case reports in dogs. Vet Surg 12:26–29, 1983; and Withrow SJ, and Holmberg DL: Mandibulectomy in the treatment of oral cancer. J Am Anim Hosp Assoc 19:273–286, 1983.

Plate 20

Approach to the Rostral Mandible

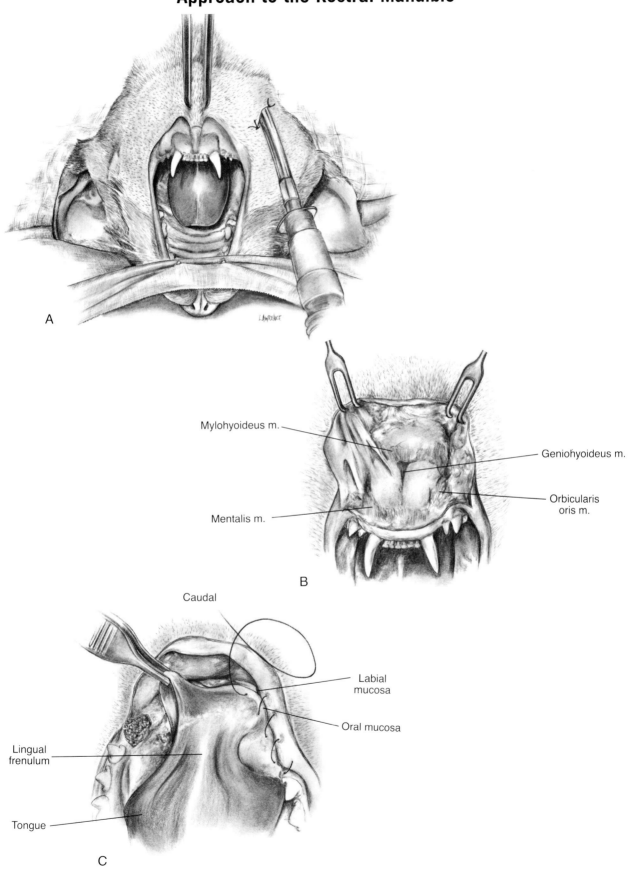

A

Mylohyoideus m.

Mentalis m.

Geniohyoideus m.

Orbicularis oris m.

B

Caudal

Labial mucosa

Oral mucosa

Lingual frenulum

Tongue

C

Approach to the Hemimandible: Feline

INDICATIONS

Neoplasia affecting the mandible that has not extensively crossed the midline.

DESCRIPTION OF THE PROCEDURE

A. The patient is positioned in lateral recumbency. The labial and oral mucosae are incised from the mandibular symphysis to the ramus of the mandible at least 1 cm peripheral to the neoplasm. The buccinator muscle is elevated from the body of the mandible using a periosteal elevator. The masseter muscle is elevated from the masseteric fossa of the mandibular ramus in similar fashion. Mandibular symphyseal osteotomy is performed using osteotome and mallet, oscillating bone saw, or bone cutters.

B. The hemimandible is displaced laterally to allow elevation of the mylohyoideus muscle from the medial mandible and the digastricus muscle from the caudoventral mandible. The mandibular alveolar artery and vein are ligated and divided near the mandibular foramen. The inferior alveolar nerve is transected. Masseter, temporalis, and pterygoideus medialis muscles are elevated from the caudal body and ramus of the mandible to expose the temporomandibular joint. The temporomandibular joint is disarticulated to complete the hemimandibulectomy.

CLOSURE

The labial and oral mucosae are apposed (Fig. **C**) using synthetic absorbable suture in a simple continuous or simple interrupted pattern.

COMMENTS

Full-thickness incision of the lip commissure, which may be performed to gain additional exposure of the caudal operative field, requires closure of oral mucosa, muscle, and skin in individual layers.

Cheiloplasty may be combined with incision of the lip commissure to shorten the commissure, preventing lateral tongue displacement as a postoperative complication.

The treatment for mucosal ulceration related to the remaining mandibular canine tooth contacting the hard palate is surgical crown shortening.

Wound dehiscence is a common complication; however, the open wound readily heals by second intention.

Food should be liquid in consistency during the first postoperative week.

Cosmesis following hemimandibulectomy is good.

Based on a procedure of Withrow SJ, and Holmberg DL: Mandibulectomy in the treatment of oral cancer. J Am Anim Hosp Assoc 19:273–286, 1983.

Plate 21

Approach to the Hemimandible

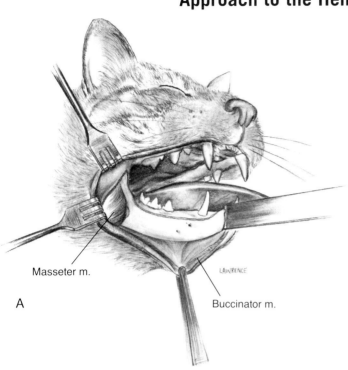

Masseter m.

Buccinator m.

A

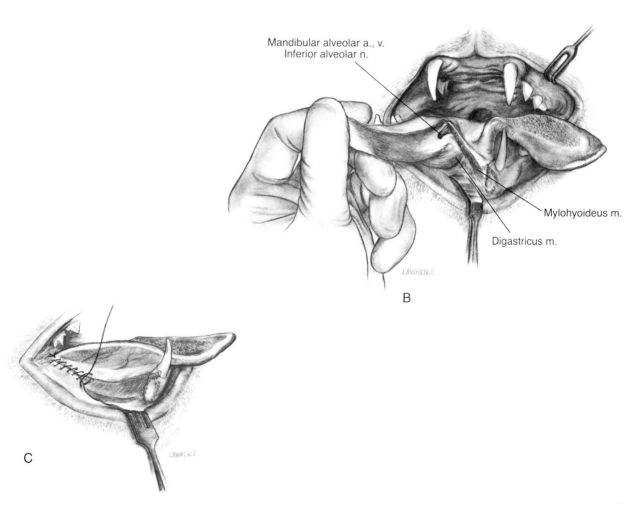

Mandibular alveolar a., v.
Inferior alveolar n.

Mylohyoideus m.

Digastricus m.

B

C

Approach to the Hard Palate

INDICATIONS

To achieve mucoperiosteum elevation for oronasal fistula repair and to aid maxillectomy closure.

DESCRIPTION OF THE PROCEDURE

A. The patient is positioned in dorsal recumbency with the neck extended. The neck is positioned over an elevated, padded area (e.g., a rolled towel) and stabilized by taping the maxilla to the operating table. The mandible is suspended to open the mouth maximally. The mucoperiosteum is incised along the palatal aspect of the rostral dental arcade. A sharp periosteal elevator is used to undermine and elevate the hard palate mucoperiosteum. The caudal limit of dissection is marked by the exit of the major palatine arteries from the major palatine foramen.

B. Hard palate mucoperiosteum may be used as a component of chronic oronasal fistula repair. Lateral and medial flaps are developed from healed perifistula tissue. The width of each flap (Figs. **A** and **B**) is one half the diameter of the fistula (inset). The flaps are inverted to provide a nasal mucosal surface. The hard palate mucoperiosteal flap is placed over the submucosal surface of the newly positioned nasal mucosa.

CLOSURE

The small perifistula flaps and hard palate mucoperiosteal flap are sutured in place using synthetic absorbable suture in simple interrupted patterns. The soft tissue defect over the hard palate heals by epithelialization.

COMMENTS

A buccal mucosal flap may be elevated and positioned to provide a nasal mucosal surface as the first layer for repair of acute oronasal fistula. The hard palate mucoperiosteal flap is used as described to provide the second, oral mucosal surface.

Based on a procedure of Nelson AW, and Wykes PM: Upper respiratory system. In *Slatter DH (ed): Textbook of Small Animal Surgery. Philadelphia, WB Saunders, 1985, pp 963–964.*

Approach to the Hard Palate

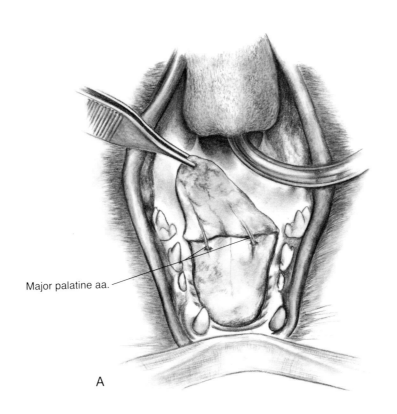

Major palatine aa.

A

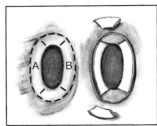

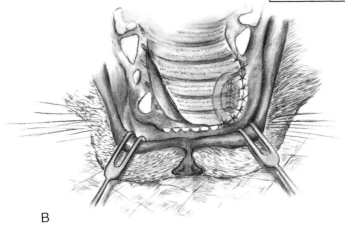

B

Approach to the Palatine Tonsil

INDICATIONS

Incisional or excisional biopsy for inflammation, neoplasia, or abnormal enlargement.

DESCRIPTION OF THE PROCEDURE

A. The patient is positioned in ventral recumbency. An open mouth is maintained using an oral speculum, and the tonsillar fossa area is examined. The edge of the tonsillar fossa is grasped with tissue forceps and retracted caudodorsally to expose the tonsil.

B. The tonsillar pedicle containing the tonsillar artery is clamped with a hemostatic forcep, and the tonsil is excised distal to the hemostat. The hemostat is removed after approximately 5 minutes, and the pedicle is examined for hemorrhage. If the pedicle bleeds, it is grasped and ligated with absorbable suture.

CLOSURE

The tonsillar fold is sutured with absorbable suture in a simple continuous pattern to prevent hemorrhage from the tonsillar fossa (inset).

COMMENTS

Hemorrhage from the operative site is the most common postoperative complication. If the tonsillar fold is sutured, hemorrhage from the tonsillar artery into the tonsillar fossa should be minimal, related to back pressure within a closed space.

Based on a procedure of Dulisch ML: The tonsils. In *Slatter DH (ed): Textbook of Small Animal Surgery. Philadelphia, WB Saunders, 1985, pp 1221–1222.*

Plate 23
Approach to the Palatine Tonsil

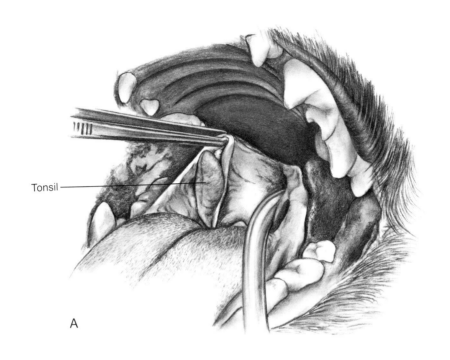

Tonsil

A

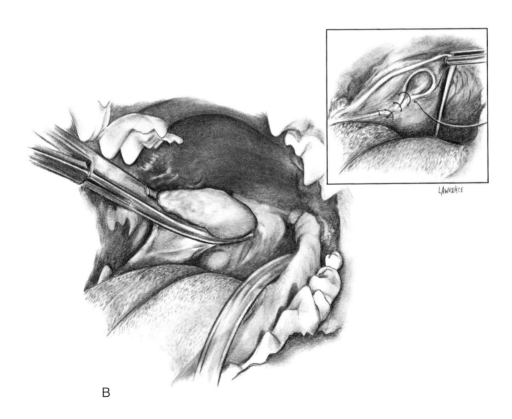

B

Head and Neck Surgery

Approach to the Hypophysis: Transoral

INDICATIONS

Hypophysectomy for patients with pituitary-dependent Cushing's disease.

DESCRIPTION OF THE PROCEDURE

A. The patient is positioned in dorsal recumbency. The neck is positioned over an elevated, padded area (e.g., a rolled towel) and stabilized by taping the maxilla to the operating table. The mandible is suspended to open the mouth maximally. A 3- to 4-cm midline incision is made in the soft palate beginning 2 cm caudal to the hamular processes and ending at the hard palate. The hamular processes are two bony protuberances of the pterygoid bone that are palpated dorsolateral to the midline.

B. A self-retaining retractor is used to maintain retraction of the soft palate. The mucoperiosteum covering the sphenoid bone is incised on the midline and reflected using a periosteal elevator. An electric hobby or air-powered drill is used to perform sphenoid osteotomy directly on the midline approximately 1 cm caudal to the intersphenoid suture. If this suture is not visualized, the osteotomy is performed on the midline 1 cm caudal to the caudal edge of the hamular processes.

Plate 24

Approach to the Hypophysis: Transoral

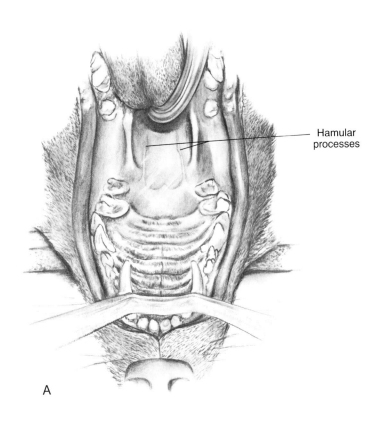

Hamular
processes

A

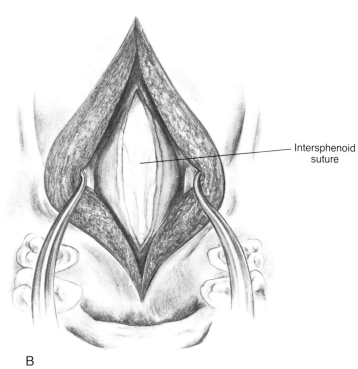

Intersphenoid
suture

B

Approach to the Hypophysis: Transoral *continued*

DESCRIPTION OF THE PROCEDURE *continued*

C. Narrow midline osteotomy will avoid the cavernous venous sinuses, which are lateral and contribute to the horseshoe configuration of the venous sinuses around the hypophysis. The inner dura mater and outer dura mater cover the hypophysis and ensheath the intercavernous and cavernous sinuses. The dural membrane is incised, and the hypophysis is removed by gentle suction. Inappropriate rostral location (rostral to the broken line) of the sphenoid osteotomy exposes the optic chiasm.

CLOSURE

Bone wax is used to fill the sphenoid osteotomy site. The soft palate is apposed using synthetic absorbable suture in simple continuous layers, including the nasopharyngeal mucosa in one layer and oropharyngeal mucosa and palatine muscles in the second layer.

COMMENTS

Trauma to the venous sinuses results in hemorrhage, which may be severe enough to inhibit completion of the procedure.

Hypophysectomy is not recommended in brachycephalic breeds owing to the increased thickness of the sphenoid bone in these animals. A transoral approach concomitant with mandibular symphysiotomy is recommended in dolichocephalic breeds.

Pituitary-dependent Cushing's disease is often managed medically using mitotane (Lysodren, Bristol Laboratories, Evansville, IN) to inhibit cortisol synthesis.

Based on a procedure of Markowitz J, Archibald J, and Downie HG: Hypophysectomy in dogs. In *Experimental Surgery. Baltimore, Williams & Wilkins, 1964, p 630.*

Plate 24
Approach to the Hypophysis: Transoral *continued*

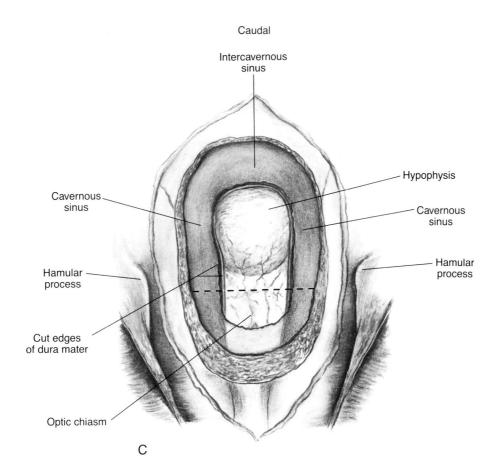

Caudal

Intercavernous
sinus

Cavernous
sinus

Hypophysis

Cavernous
sinus

Hamular
process

Hamular
process

Cut edges
of dura mater

Optic chiasm

C

Approach to the Oropharynx

INDICATIONS

Pharyngotomy for placement of feeding tube or endotracheal tube.

DESCRIPTION OF THE PROCEDURE

A. The patient is positioned in lateral recumbency and the neck is extended. The surgeon's finger or an angled forcep is used to provide medial-to-lateral pressure from within the oropharynx between the ramus of the mandible and the epihyoid bone. A skin incision is made over this area and continued through the platysma muscle. The sphincter colli muscle is displaced or separated, followed by pharyngotomy using sharp incision over an instrument or puncture with a hemostat.

B. The distal end of the feeding or endotracheal tube is passed through the pharyngotomy and placed into the esophagus or trachea, respectively.

CLOSURE

The contaminated pharyngotomy site is allowed to heal by second intention, regardless of the duration of tube placement.

COMMENTS

Modification of this technique for feeding tube placement has been advocated to theoretically decrease the risk of food aspiration resulting from tube interference with the epiglottis. The modification involves placement of the tube in the dorsal pharynx caudal to the epihyoid bone. Alternatives to pharyngotomy for feeding tube placement include nasoesophageal intubation, tube gastrostomy, and endoscopic guided percutaneous tube gastrostomy.

Endotracheal tube placement via pharyngotomy may be advantageous when extensive surgery of the oral cavity is planned.

Based on a procedure of Bohning RH, DeHoff WD, McElihinney A, et al: Pharyngostomy for maintenance of the anorectic animal. J Am Vet Med Assoc 156:611–615, 1970.

Plate 25

Approach to the Oropharynx

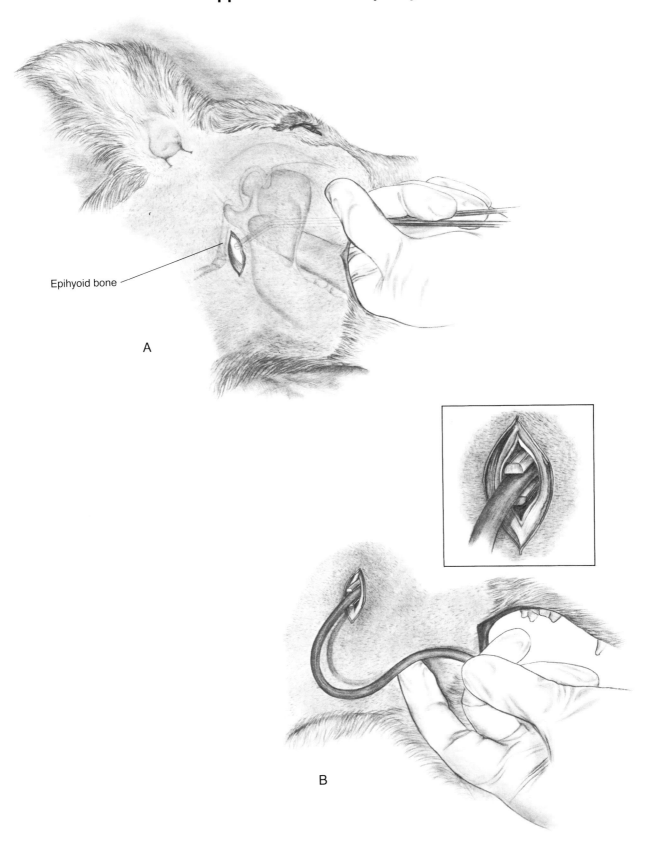

Epihyoid bone

A

B

Approach to the Mandibular and Sublingual Salivary Glands

INDICATIONS

Resective surgery for treatment of cervical, pharyngeal, and sublingual mucoceles and salivary gland neoplasia.

DESCRIPTION OF THE PROCEDURE

A. The patient is positioned in lateral recumbency. The patient's neck is rotated contralaterally, extended over an elevated padded area (e.g., a rolled towel), and the mandible is secured to the operating table using adhesive tape. A curvilinear skin incision is made from the bifurcation of the external jugular vein to the caudoventral aspect of the body of the mandible.

B. Subcutaneous tissue and platysma muscle are incised, followed by division of the parotidoauricularis muscle to expose glandular, venous, and neurologic structures.

Plate 26

Approach to the Mandibular and Sublingual Salivary Glands

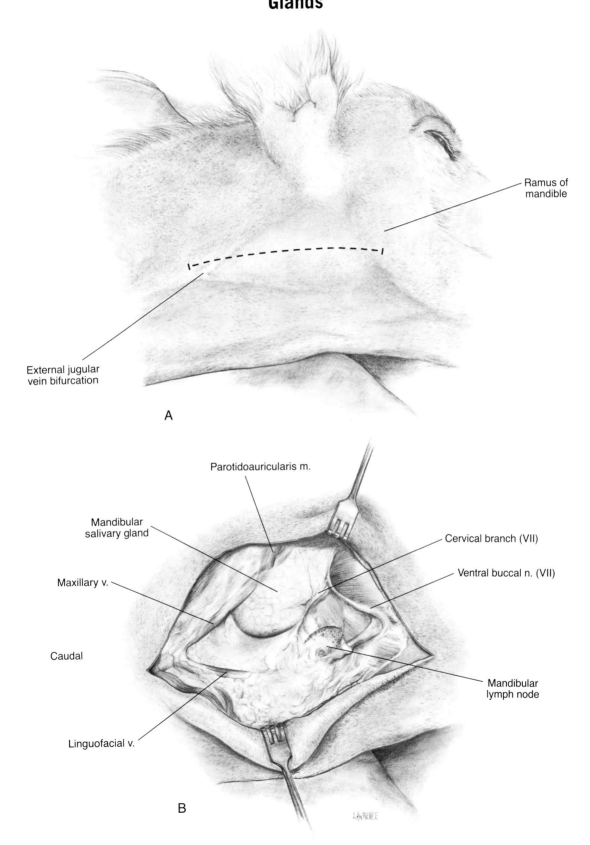

Ramus of mandible

External jugular vein bifurcation

A

Parotidoauricularis m.

Mandibular salivary gland

Maxillary v.

Caudal

Linguofacial v.

Cervical branch (VII)

Ventral buccal n. (VII)

Mandibular lymph node

B

Approach to the Mandibular and Sublingual Salivary Glands *continued*

DESCRIPTION OF THE PROCEDURE *continued*

C. The mandibular salivary gland is identified between the maxillary and linguofacial veins. Its capsule is incised, and the gland parenchyma is grasped with tissue forceps to provide caudal traction. The fascia is incised between the masseter and digastricus muscles, allowing digital and sharp dissection of connective tissue attachments to expose the entire mandibular salivary gland and the contiguous sublingual gland complex. The end point for dissection is visualization of the lingual nerve, which courses laterally over the sublingual salivary gland complex. The gland-duct complex is ligated and divided just caudal to the lingual nerve.

D. The digastricus muscle may obscure the surgeon's view rostrally, necessitating either increased caudal retraction on the mandibular and sublingual gland complex or manipulation of the complex under the digastricus muscle and floor of the mucocele to allow further rostral dissection. The mucocele can be incised and drained to facilitate tissue manipulation around the digastricus muscle. Alternatively, myotomy of the digastricus muscle can be performed to aid complete visualization of the gland-duct complex and the location of the defect causing mucocele.

CLOSURE

Soft latex drains (Penrose) are placed through the mucocele and maintained for 1 to 3 days to allow drainage. The digastricus muscle, if incised, should be apposed with synthetic absorbable suture using a mattress pattern. Subcutaneous tissues are apposed with similar material in a simple interrupted pattern followed by skin closure using nonabsorbable suture in a simple interrupted pattern.

COMMENT

Blood vessels that supply the mandibular salivary gland are encountered on the dorsomedial aspect of the gland and should be cauterized or ligated.

The gland-duct defect causing mucocele rarely occurs rostral to the lingual nerve. If the lingual nerve is not visualized, dissection may continue to the oral mucosa. The surgeon should make every effort to isolate the origin of the defect, verifying that the correct side has been operated. Failure to identify the defect indicates that the mucocele may have originated from the contralateral gland-duct complex. In the authors' experience, bilateral resection of the mandibular and sublingual gland-duct complex is not associated with xerostomia.

The mandibular lymph node should be differentiated from salivary tissue.

This procedure is recommended for cervical, pharyngeal, and sublingual mucoceles, because defect location is variable and the mandibular and sublingual glands are closely associated.

Based on a procedure of Spreull JSA, and Head KW: Cervical salivary cysts in the dog. J Sm Anim Pract 8:17–35, 1967.

Plate 26

Approach to the Mandibular and Sublingual Salivary Glands *continued*

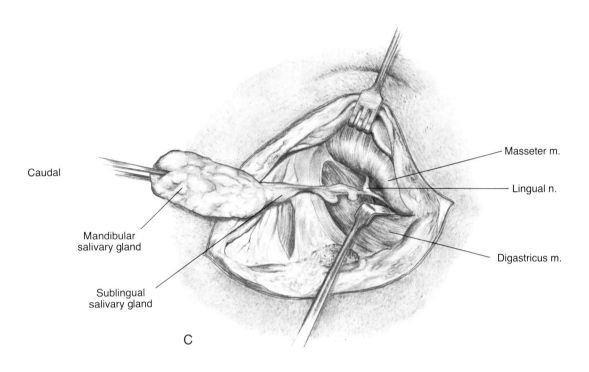

Caudal

Masseter m.

Lingual n.

Mandibular
salivary gland

Digastricus m.

Sublingual
salivary gland

C

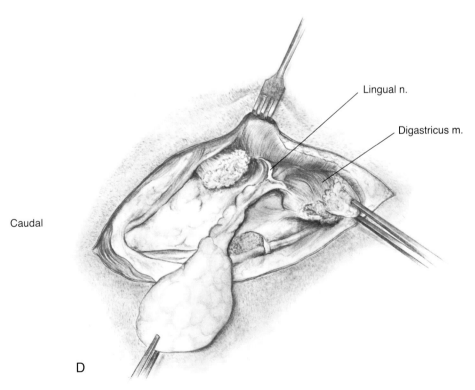

Lingual n.

Digastricus m.

Caudal

D

Approach to the Parotid Salivary Gland

INDICATIONS

Resective surgery for treatment of parotid salivary gland neoplasia and incisional biopsy.

DESCRIPTION OF THE PROCEDURE

A. The patient is positioned in lateral recumbency. A skin incision is made from the dorsal vertical ear canal to a point midway between the ramus of the mandible and the bifurcation of the jugular vein.

B. The platysma muscle is incised to expose the origin of the parotidoauricularis muscle, vertical ear canal, and parotid salivary gland. The parotidoauricularis muscle is incised at its origin and retracted. The caudal auricular vein is ligated and divided.

Plate 27
Approach to the Parotid Salivary Gland

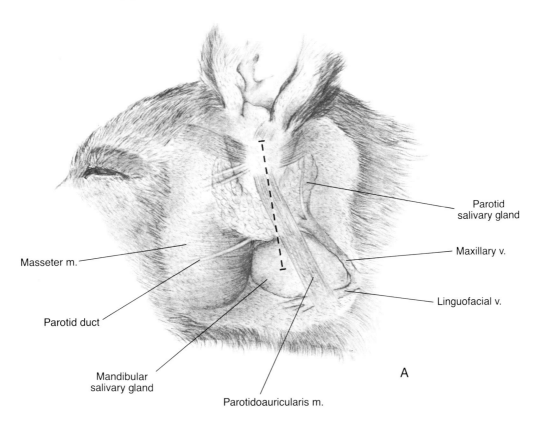

Masseter m.

Parotid duct

Mandibular
salivary gland

Parotidoauricularis m.

Parotid
salivary gland

Maxillary v.

Linguofacial v.

A

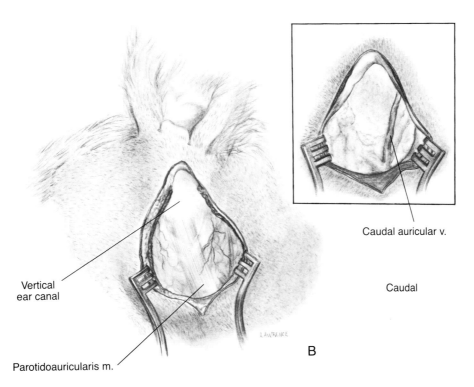

Vertical
ear canal

Parotidoauricularis m.

Caudal auricular v.

Caudal

B

Approach to the Parotid Salivary Gland *continued*

DESCRIPTION OF THE PROCEDURE *continued*

C. The V-shaped parotid salivary gland is resected beginning at its dorsocaudal angle. The ventral angle of the parotid salivary gland is contiguous with the mandibular salivary gland. The plane of dissection continues between these two glands, exposing the maxillary vein, which is ligated and divided.

D. The plane of dissection is continued between the vertical ear canal and the gland. The facial nerve should be visualized and avoided as it courses near the junction of the vertical and horizontal ear canals. Branches of the facial nerve should be dissected from the deep portion of the gland ventral to the external ear canal toward the dorsorostral angle. The superficial temporal vein courses through the gland as a tributary of the maxillary vein, necessitating its ligation and division. The parotid duct is resected and ligated as it exits the parenchyma of the gland.

CLOSURE

The incision in the parotidoauricularis muscle may be closed with fine synthetic absorbable suture in a simple interrupted pattern. Subcutaneous tissues are apposed with similar material in a simple interrupted pattern followed by skin closure using nonabsorbable suture in a simple interrupted pattern.

COMMENTS

The parotid artery and tributaries from other regional arteries supply the gland. These vessels usually enter the gland from the medial aspect and should be cauterized or ligated and divided, depending on their size. Venous structures seem to predominate in this area.

Placement of a Penrose drain may be indicated if there is substantial dead space following resection.

Neoplasia of this gland may increase vascular supply to the area and distort normal anatomy, inhibiting visualization of vital structures. Curative surgery would be unlikely. Radiation therapy should be considered as a primary or adjunctive treatment option.

Plate 27

Approach to the Parotid Salivary Gland *continued*

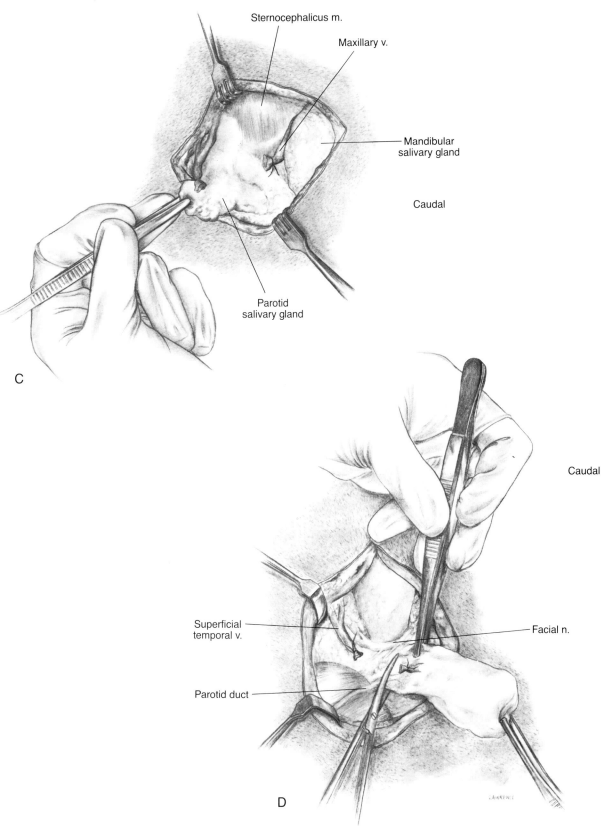

Sternocephalicus m.

Maxillary v.

Mandibular
salivary gland

Caudal

Parotid
salivary gland

C

Caudal

Superficial
temporal v.

Facial n.

Parotid duct

D

Approach to the Parotid Salivary Gland Duct

INDICATIONS

Parotid duct transposition for treatment of keratoconjunctivitis sicca refractory to medical management.

DESCRIPTION OF THE PROCEDURE

A. The patient is positioned in lateral recumbency. The parotid duct opens into the oral cavity at the rostral end of a small buccal mucosal papilla opposite the caudal aspect of the maxillary fourth premolar. The papilla is located and instrumented with a blunt-tipped, 21-gauge catheter or cannula to aid dissection and traction on the duct. A circumferential mucosal incision is made around the papilla, including a 0.5-cm cuff of buccal mucosa (inset). The catheter helps prevent iatrogenic trauma to the duct during sharp submucosal dissection to isolate its rostral aspect. Traction on the mucosa and catheter facilitates subcutaneous sharp and blunt dissection to mobilize the duct from its location in superficial fascia on the lateral surface of the masseter muscle.

B. The ocular portion of the procedure begins with a 1.5-cm incision in the ventrolateral conjunctival fornix. A hemostat is used to develop a subcutaneous tunnel between the fornix and the previously dissected area on the lateral masseter muscle. The catheter is removed, and a stay suture is applied to the cuff of buccal mucosal tissue surrounding the papilla. The suture is grasped by the hemostat placed through the oral incision. The papilla is transposed to the ventrolateral conjunctival fornix and sutured to the ocular incision (inset).

CLOSURE

The buccal mucosa surrounding the papilla is apposed to the conjunctiva using synthetic absorbable suture in a simple interrupted pattern. The oral wound is allowed to heal by second intention.

COMMENTS

The catheter may be replaced in the parotid duct during or following suture placement to ensure duct patency. Alternatively, a fine-gauge stay suture may be used to attach the catheter hub to the buccal mucosal cuff at the beginning of the procedure to prevent the duct from twisting.

The procedure may be performed "open" by skin incision over the duct as it courses on the lateral aspect of the masseter muscle, providing visualization of the duct during dissection.

All available medical therapy should be tried before surgery is performed on patients with keratoconjunctivitis sicca.

Based on a procedure of Jensen HE: Keratitis sicca and parotid duct transposition. Comp Contin Educ Pract Vet 1:721–726, 1979.

Plate 28

Approach to the Parotid Salivary Gland Duct

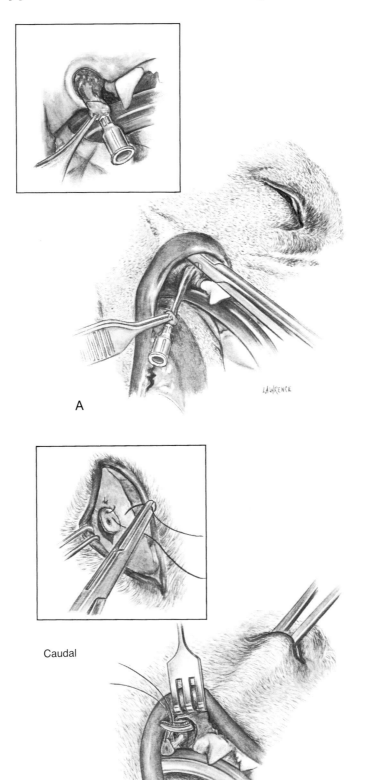

A

Caudal

B

Approach to the Zygomatic Salivary Gland

INDICATIONS

Resective surgery for treatment of zygomatic salivary gland neoplasia and mucocele.

DESCRIPTION OF THE PROCEDURE

A. The patient is positioned in lateral recumbency. A skin incision is made over the dorsal rim of the zygomatic arch.

B. The periorbital fascia and the zygomatic periosteum are incised and retracted dorsally. Periorbital fat is removed using sharp dissection (inset). The zygomatic gland is visualized ventral to the periorbital fat.

C. Partial ostectomy of the zygomatic arch using bone rongeurs is usually required to achieve additional exposure. An anastomotic branch between the deep facial and external ophthalmic veins is observed ventrally and should be avoided. Zygomatic salivary tissue is friable, allowing removal by blunt dissection and traction on the gland with tissue forceps.

CLOSURE

The periorbital fascia is apposed using synthetic absorbable suture in a simple interrupted pattern. The skin is apposed with absorbable suture in a continuous pattern in the subcutaneous or subcuticular area, avoiding the use of skin sutures that may irritate periocular tissues.

COMMENTS

The orbital ligament may be incised to increase exposure of the operative field. Neoplastic disease may require resection of the entire zygomatic arch for exposure. Resected bone should not be replaced, so that the opportunity for tumor-free tissue margins can be maximized. Partial resection of the zygomatic arch is associated with normal function and good cosmesis.

Based on a procedure of Spreull JSA, and Archibald J: Glands of the head and neck. In *Archibald J (ed): Canine Surgery. Santa Barbara, CA, American Veterinary Publications, 1974, pp 274–276.*

Plate 29
Approach to the Zygomatic Salivary Gland

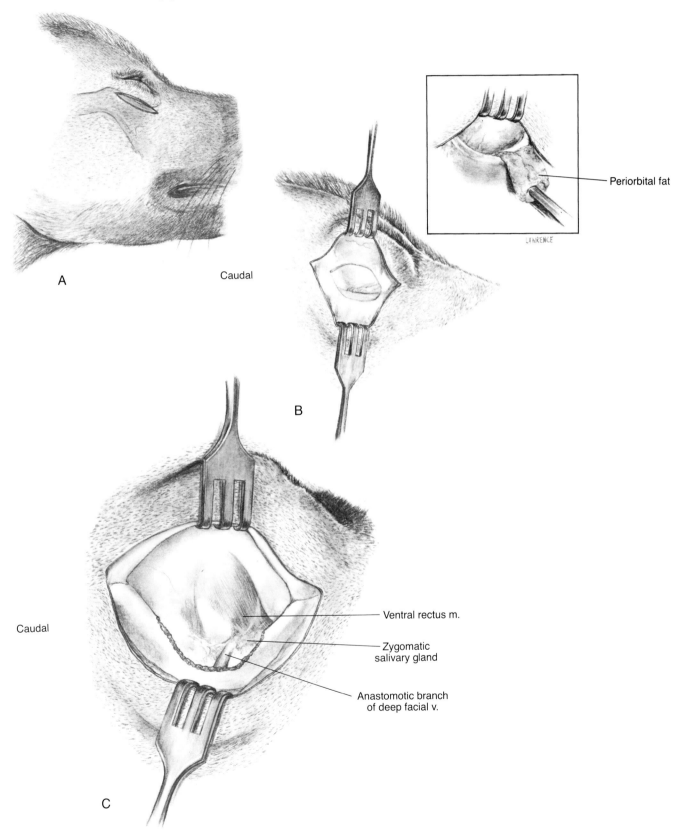

A

Caudal

Periorbital fat

LAWRENCE

B

Caudal

Ventral rectus m.

Zygomatic
salivary gland

Anastomotic branch
of deep facial v.

C

Approach to the Proximal Esophagus

INDICATIONS

Cricopharyngeal myotomy for cricopharyngeal stage dysphagia and exploratory surgery for perforation of the esophagus by a foreign body.

DESCRIPTION OF THE PROCEDURE

A. The patient is positioned in right lateral recumbency. The neck is positioned over an elevated, padded area (e.g., a rolled towel), rotated to the right with elevation of the left mandible, and stabilized by taping the maxilla to the operating table. A skin incision begins at the caudal angle of the mandible and continues caudally approximately 8 cm over the dorsolateral aspect of the larynx.

B. The platysma and parotidoauricularis muscles are incised. The sternocephalicus muscle and jugular vein are retracted dorsally, and the sternohyoideus muscle is retracted ventrally to expose the laryngeal area.

Plate 30
Approach to the Proximal Esophagus

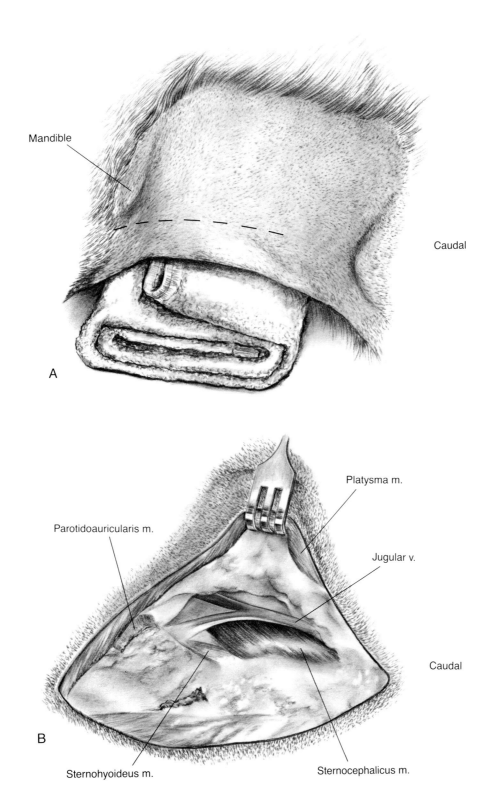

Mandible

Caudal

A

Parotidoauricularis m.

Platysma m.

Jugular v.

Caudal

B

Sternohyoideus m.

Sternocephalicus m.

Approach to the Proximal Esophagus *continued*

DESCRIPTION OF THE PROCEDURE *continued*

C. The thyroid cartilage is palpated, and loose areolar tissue over the area is dissected to expose the sternothyroideus, cricothyroideus, and thyrohyoideus muscles at their attachment to the thyroid cartilage. Small pharyngeal and cricothyroid branches of the cranial thyroid artery may be incised and cauterized to provide hemostasis. Areolar tissue near the thyroid gland may be visualized between the trachea and the sternothyroideus muscle.

D. The retractor is repositioned on the sternothyroideus muscle, allowing the larynx to be rotated ventrally 90° to expose the cricopharyngeus and thyropharyngeus muscles. Alternatively, a stay suture may be placed in the thyroid cartilage to aid laryngeal rotation.

E. Myotomy of the cricopharyngeus and thyropharyngeus muscles is performed midway between the median raphe and their origin. Placement of a tube in the esophagus aids its identification and the development of a dissection plane between the muscles and the esophagus.

CLOSURE

Subcutaneous tissues are apposed using synthetic absorbable suture in a simple interrupted pattern. Skin is apposed using synthetic nonabsorbable suture in the same pattern.

COMMENTS

The authors recommend concurrent myotomy of the thyropharyngeus muscle, because this muscle may also contribute to cricopharyngeal phase dysphagia. Myotomy may be performed within the muscle laterally or on the dorsal median raphe.

Accidental perforation of the esophagus should be repaired with synthetic absorbable suture in a simple interrupted pattern. The size of perforation affects postoperative feeding guidelines or the decision to provide a feeding tube to bypass the upper esophagus.

Partial myectomy of the cricopharyngeus and thyropharyngeus muscles is advocated by some surgeons to decrease the possibility of fibrous stricture associated with myotomy healing.

Based on a procedure of Sokolovsky V: Cricopharyngeal achalasia in a dog. J Am Vet Med Assoc 151:281–283, 1967.

Plate 30

Approach to the Proximal Esophagus *continued*

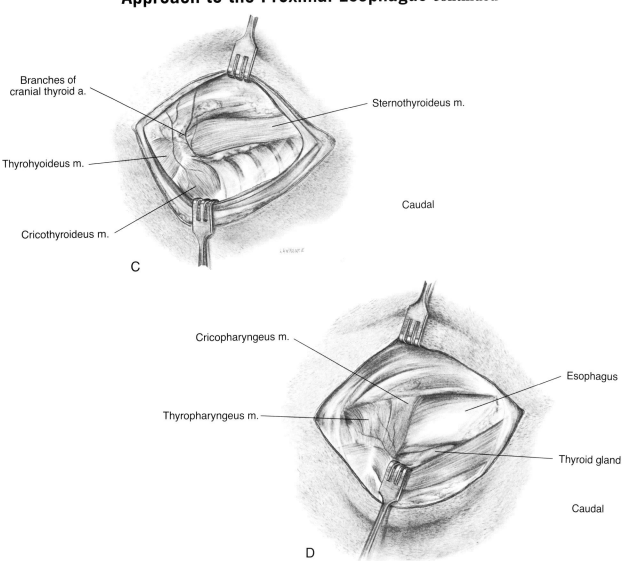

Branches of
cranial thyroid a.

Sternothyroideus m.

Thyrohyoideus m.

Caudal

Cricothyroideus m.

C

Cricopharyngeus m.

Esophagus

Thyropharyngeus m.

Thyroid gland

Caudal

D

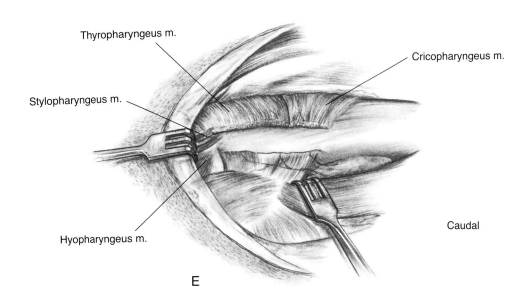

Thyropharyngeus m.

Cricopharyngeus m.

Stylopharyngeus m.

Hyopharyngeus m.

Caudal

E

Approach to the Thyroid and Parathyroid Glands: Canine

INDICATIONS

Neoplasia of the thyroid and parathyroid glands.

DESCRIPTION OF THE PROCEDURE

A. The patient is positioned in dorsal recumbency. The patient's neck is extended over an elevated padded area (e.g., a rolled towel), and the head is secured to the operating table using adhesive tape. A ventral midline skin incision is made from the caudal larynx to a location 2 to 3 cm cranial to the manubrium.

B. Following incision of the platysma muscle and the subcutaneous tissues, the paired sternohyoideus muscles are divided along midline. Caudal extension of the incision requires division of the sternocephalicus muscles. The sternohyoideus and sterno-thyroideus muscles are retracted to expose the trachea. Ligation and division or electrocoagulation of one or more of the caudal thyroid veins is usually required.

Plate 31

Approach to the Thyroid and Parathyroid Glands: Canine

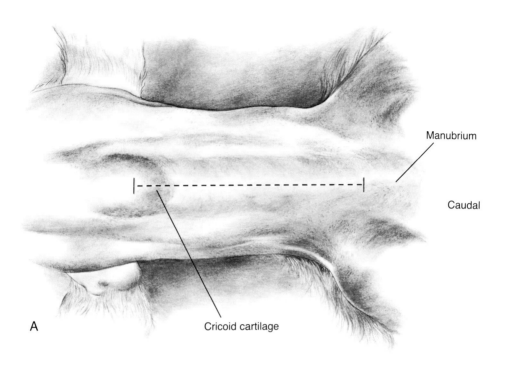

Manubrium

Caudal

Cricoid cartilage

A

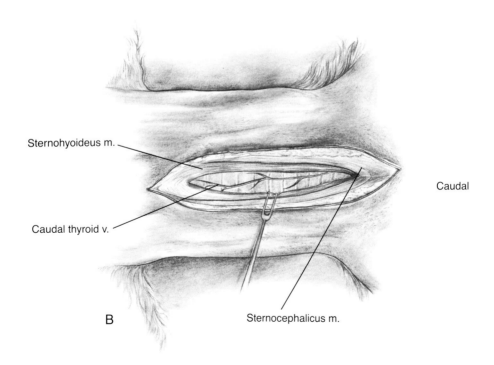

Sternohyoideus m.

Caudal thyroid v.

Sternocephalicus m.

Caudal

B

Approach to the Thyroid and Parathyroid Glands: Canine *continued*

DESCRIPTION OF THE PROCEDURE *continued*

C. Division of the paired sternohyoideus muscles along the ventral larynx coupled with lateral retraction allows visualization of the thyroid gland. The external parathyroid gland may be visualized near the cranial pole of the thyroid gland. The glands are located in deep cervical fascia adjacent to the trachea and caudal to the cricoid cartilage.

D. The left thyroid gland is located further caudally than the right thyroid gland, between the third and eighth tracheal rings. This gland has the same vascular supply as the right; however, the components of the carotid sheath are displaced by the esophagus and do not come in contact with the gland.

Plate 31

Approach to the Thyroid and Parathyroid Glands:
Canine *continued*

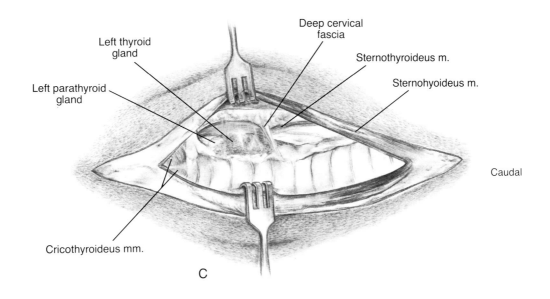

Left thyroid gland

Deep cervical fascia

Sternothyroideus m.

Sternohyoideus m.

Left parathyroid gland

Caudal

Cricothyroideus mm.

C

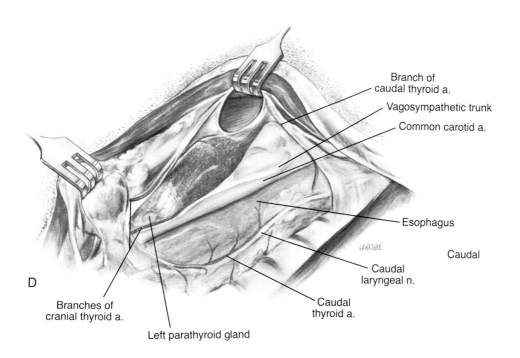

Branch of caudal thyroid a.

Vagosympathetic trunk

Common carotid a.

Esophagus

Caudal

Caudal laryngeal n.

D

Branches of cranial thyroid a.

Left parathyroid gland

Caudal thyroid a.

LAWRENCE

Approach to the Thyroid and Parathyroid Glands: Canine *continued*

DESCRIPTION OF THE PROCEDURE *continued*

E. The deep cervical fascia and the proper fascia of the trachea are incised to expose the vascular supply to the right thyroid and parathyroid glands. The cranial and caudal thyroid arteries and veins provide blood to these glands. During thyroidectomy, these vessels must be cauterized or ligated and divided near the capsule of the thyroid gland, while blood supply to the external parathyroid gland is preserved. A sterile cotton applicator facilitates meticulous dissection in this area, allowing appropriate hemostasis for extracapsular dissection and removal of the entire thyroid gland, including the internal parathyroid gland.

CLOSURE

The sternohyoideus and the sternocephalicus muscles are apposed using synthetic absorbable suture in a simple interrupted pattern. Subcutaneous tissues are closed similarly, followed by skin apposition using nonabsorbable suture in a simple interrupted pattern.

COMMENTS

Thyroid neoplasia in dogs is usually diagnosed when the neoplasm is relatively large and after local metastasis. It is associated with extensive neovascularization requiring strict hemostasis. Adjacent structures including the esophagus, the recurrent laryngeal nerve, the carotid artery, the jugular vein, and the vagosympathetic trunk may be involved. Curative surgery is unlikely, warranting a guarded prognosis and a recommendation of postoperative adjuvant therapy.

Removal of the parathyroid gland for neoplasia requires a similar surgical approach. If the external parathyroid gland is affected, it is dissected from the thyroid capsule, with vascular supply to the cranial aspect of the thyroid gland preserved. If the internal parathyroid gland is affected, it is removed as a component of thyroidectomy, as described earlier in this discussion.

The clinician should consider postoperative treatment for hormonal imbalances causing hypocalcemia related to parathyroidectomy and for hypothyroidism in patients undergoing bilateral thyroidectomy.

The right thyroid gland is bordered dorsolaterally by the common carotid artery, the internal jugular vein, and the vagosympathetic trunk. These structures are normally not intimately associated with the thyroid gland. The right recurrent laryngeal nerve, however, requires identification and manipulation during thyroidectomy as it courses along the dorsal aspect of the right thyroid gland.

Based on a procedure of Schotthauer CF: The thyroid gland. In Mayer K, LaCroix JV, and Hoskins HP (eds): Canine Surgery. Santa Barbara, CA, American Veterinary Publications, 1957, pp 389–390.

Plate 31

Approach to the Thyroid and Parathyroid Glands:
Canine *continued*

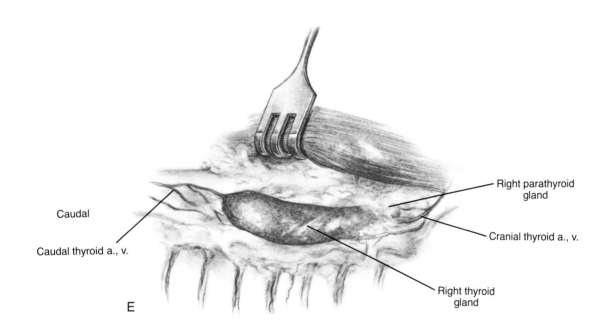

Caudal

Caudal thyroid a., v.

Right parathyroid gland

Cranial thyroid a., v.

Right thyroid gland

E

Approach to the Thyroid and Parathyroid Glands: Feline

INDICATIONS

Neoplasia of the thyroid and parathyroid glands.

DESCRIPTION OF THE PROCEDURE

A. The patient is positioned in dorsal recumbency. The patient's neck is extended over an elevated padded area (e.g., a rolled towel), and the head is secured to the operating table using adhesive tape. A ventral midline skin incision is made from the caudal larynx to a location 2 to 3 cm cranial to the manubrium.

Plate 32
Approach to the Thyroid and Parathyroid Glands: Feline

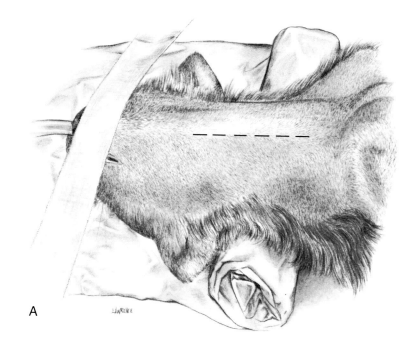

A

Approach to the Thyroid and Parathyroid Glands: Feline *continued*

DESCRIPTION OF THE PROCEDURE *continued*

B. The paired sternohyoideus muscles are separated on midline and with the sterno-thyroideus muscles are lateralized with self-retaining retractors. The thyroid and parathyroid glands are observed in a caudal, midtracheal position, in contrast to the more cranial location of these glands in the dog. The external parathyroid gland may be visualized near the cranial pole of the thyroid gland. The cranial thyroid artery supplies the thyroid and parathyroid glands. This vessel must be cauterized or ligated and divided near the capsule of the thyroid gland, with blood supply to the parathyroid gland preserved.

C. Extracapsular dissection and removal of the entire thyroid gland and its capsule, including the internal parathyroid gland, may jeopardize vascular supply to the external parathyroid gland. A sterile cotton applicator facilitates meticulous intra-capsular dissection, which preserves the thyroid gland capsule in this area, allowing appropriate hemostasis and ensuring preservation of vascular supply to the external parathyroid gland. The cranial and caudal thyroid veins drain the surgical area and may be cauterized or ligated to achieve hemostasis, depending on the surgical technique (intra- or extracapsular dissection).

CLOSURE

The sternohyoideus muscles are apposed using synthetic absorbable suture in a simple interrupted pattern. Subcutaneous tissues are closed similarly, followed by skin apposition using nonabsorbable suture in a simple interrupted pattern.

COMMENTS

Thyroidectomy is most commonly performed for hyperthyroidism in cats. Because bilateral disease is common, bilateral thyroidectomy is recommended.

Removal of the parathyroid gland for neoplasia requires a similar surgical approach. If the external parathyroid gland is affected, it is dissected from the thyroid capsule, with vascular supply to the cranial aspect of the thyroid gland preserved. If the internal parathyroid gland is affected, it is removed as a component of thyroidectomy, as described earlier in this discussion.

The clinician should consider postoperative treatment for hormonal imbalances causing hypocalcemia related to parathyroidectomy and for hypothyroidism in patients undergoing bilateral thyroidectomy.

The intracapsular dissection technique risks incomplete removal of adenomatous thyroid tissue, which may cause recurrence of hyperthyroidism. The authors prefer the extra-capsular dissection technique so that this potential complication can be prevented.

Based on a procedure of Schotthauer CF: The thyroid gland. In Mayer K, LaCroix JV, and Hoskins HP (eds): Canine Surgery. Santa Barbara, CA, American Veterinary Publications, 1957, pp 389–390.

Plate 32

Approach to the Thyroid and Parathyroid Glands:
Feline *continued*

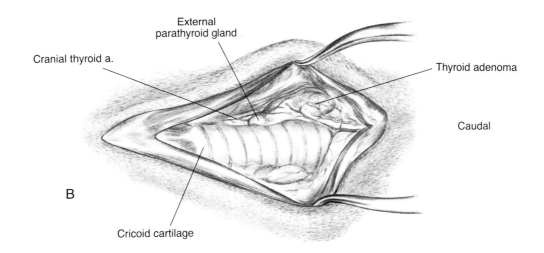

External
parathyroid gland

Cranial thyroid a.

Thyroid adenoma

Caudal

Cricoid cartilage

B

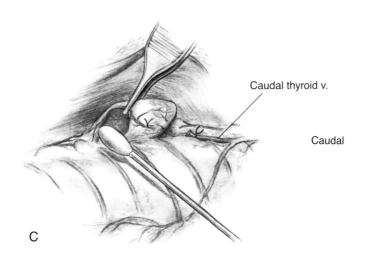

Caudal thyroid v.

Caudal

C

Approach to the Ventral Tympanic Bulla: Canine

INDICATIONS

Exploratory surgery of the tympanic bulla for incisional biopsy, microbial culture, and/or ventral drainage and lavage in patients with otitis media.

DESCRIPTION OF THE PROCEDURE

A. The patient is positioned in dorsal recumbency. The patient's neck is extended over an elevated padded area (e.g., a rolled towel), and the head is secured to the operating table using adhesive tape. A paramedian skin incision is made 2 cm lateral to the midline. It extends from the level of the bifurcation of the jugular vein to a level even with the midbody of the mandible. The incision is centered on a line perpendicular to the midline at the ramus of the mandible.

B. The incision is continued through subcutaneous tissues and platysma muscle to venous structures and the digastricus muscle. The mylohyoideus muscle, which courses dorsal and perpendicular to the digastricus muscle, is incised along its caudal aspect to expose the lingual vein.

Plate 33

Approach to the Ventral Tympanic Bulla: Canine

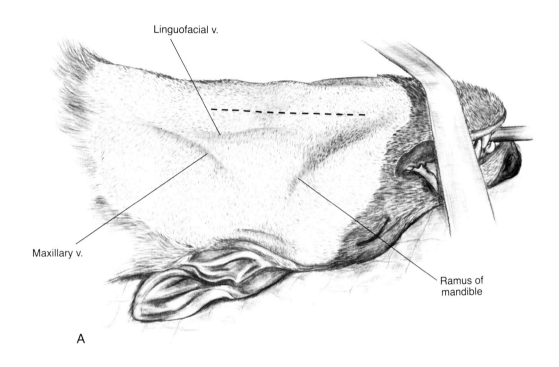

Linguofacial v.

Maxillary v.

Ramus of
mandible

A

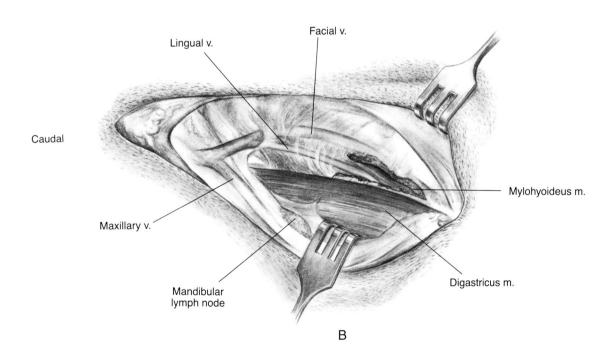

Facial v.

Lingual v.

Caudal

Maxillary v.

Mandibular
lymph node

Mylohyoideus m.

Digastricus m.

B

Approach to the Ventral Tympanic Bulla: Canine *continued*

DESCRIPTION OF THE PROCEDURE *continued*

C. The mylohyoideus and digastricus muscles are retracted to expose the hypoglossal nerve and the lingual artery medial to the styloglossus muscle and lateral to the hyoglossus and hyopharyngeus muscles.

D. The plane of dissection is continued dorsally along the medial aspect of the hypoglossal nerve and the lingual artery. The ventral tympanic bulla is palpated caudal to the stylohyoid bone. The tympanic bulla is bordered by the pterygoideus medialis muscle cranially and the longus capitis muscle medially. The external carotid artery and the communicating rami of the glossopharyngeal nerve are visualized and avoided. Fascia and thin muscle fibers are elevated from the ventral aspect of the tympanic bulla using a periosteal elevator. An intramedullary pin or bone trephine may be used to perform bulla osteotomy, followed by additional bone removal with rongeurs.

CLOSURE

A drain system may be placed to allow postoperative drainage and/or lavage of the middle ear. The mylohyoideus muscle, the digastricus fascia, and the subcutaneous tissues are apposed in individual layers with synthetic absorbable suture in simple interrupted patterns. Skin is apposed using synthetic nonabsorbable suture in a simple interrupted pattern.

COMMENTS

The inner ear, located dorsomedially, should be avoided during exploration and curettage. Disruption of this area may lead to a hearing deficiency and damage to neurologic structures, including the vestibulocochlear and facial nerves and the vagosympathetic trunk. Neurologic deficit related to injury of these structures (e.g., head tilt, facial paralysis, and Horner's syndrome) is usually transient if the insult is minor.

Based on a procedure of McNutt GW, and McCoy JE: Bulla osteotomy in the dog. J Am Vet Med Assoc 77:617–620, 1930.

Plate 33

Approach to the Ventral Tympanic Bulla:
Canine *continued*

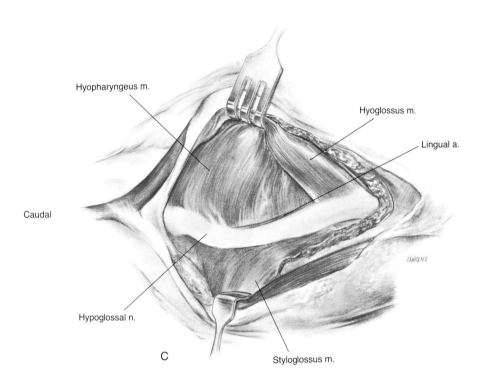

Hyopharyngeus m.

Hyoglossus m.

Lingual a.

Caudal

Hypoglossal n.

Styloglossus m.

C

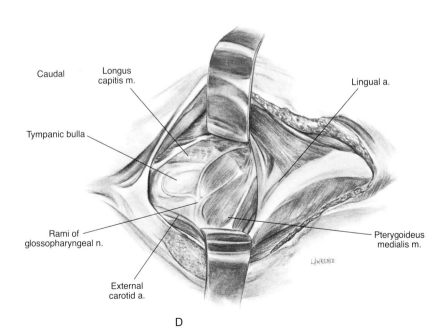

Caudal

Longus capitis m.

Lingual a.

Tympanic bulla

Rami of glossopharyngeal n.

Pterygoideus medialis m.

External carotid a.

D

Approach to the Ventral Tympanic Bulla: Feline

INDICATIONS

Exploratory surgery of the tympanic bulla for incisional biopsy, microbial culture, and ventral drainage and/or lavage in patients with otitis media and as a component of treatment for nasopharyngeal polyp.

DESCRIPTION OF THE PROCEDURE

A. The patient is positioned in dorsal recumbency. The patient's neck is extended over an elevated padded area (e.g., a rolled towel), and the head is secured to the operating table using adhesive tape. A paramedian skin incision is made 2 cm lateral to the midline between the proximal trachea and the most caudal aspect of the mandible. It extends from the level of the bifurcation of the jugular vein to a level even with the midbody of the mandible. The incision is centered on a line perpendicular to the midline at the ramus of the mandible.

B. The incision is continued through the subcutaneous tissues and the platysma muscle. Dissection continues between the linguofacial and maxillary veins as they converge to form the external jugular vein. The mandibular salivary gland is retracted laterally, and the fascia between the masseter and digastricus muscles is incised. Dorsal digital palpation aids identification of the ventral tympanic bulla and the stylohyoid bone.

Plate 34

Approach to the Ventral Tympanic Bulla: Feline

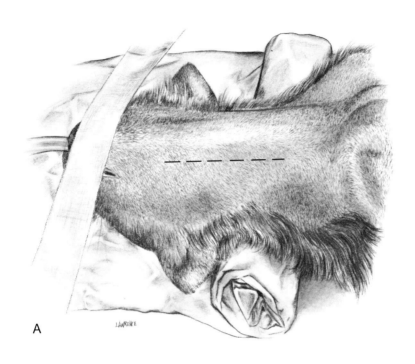

A

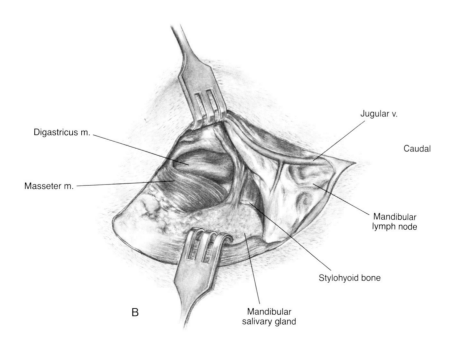

Digastricus m.

Masseter m.

Jugular v.

Caudal

Mandibular
lymph node

Stylohyoid bone

Mandibular
salivary gland

B

Approach to the Ventral Tympanic Bulla: Feline *continued*

DESCRIPTION OF THE PROCEDURE *continued*

C. Medial retraction of the digastricus muscle and lateral retraction of the salivary gland tissue allows visualization of the ventral tympanic bulla. Structures that should be identified in the dorsal operative field include the hypoglossal nerve, the lingual artery, the stylohyoid bone, and the styloglossus muscle.

D. Neurovascular structures ventral to the tympanic bulla are retracted, and an intramedullary pin or bone trephine may be used to perform bulla osteotomy, followed by additional bone removal with rongeurs. The ventromedial and dorsolateral compartments of the tympanic bulla are explored, avoiding sympathetic nerve supply to the eye.

CLOSURE

Ventral drainage techniques may be applied if indicated, followed by apposition of fascia between the digastricus and masseter muscles using synthetic absorbable suture in a simple interrupted pattern. Subcutaneous tissues are apposed similarly, followed by skin closure using synthetic nonabsorbable suture in a simple interrupted pattern.

COMMENTS

Medial retraction of the digastricus muscle protects neurovascular structures ventral to the tympanic bulla. Alternatively, dissection may be performed in the plane medial to the digastricus muscle.

Compartmentalization of the tympanic bulla is unique to the cat. Ventral bulla osteotomy usually exposes only the ventromedial compartment. Thorough exploration requires the surgeon to use bone rongeurs to remove the bony septum that separates the two compartments. This is especially important in cats with inflammatory nasopharyngeal polyp, which often is present in the dorsolateral compartment only.

Patients may have clinical signs of Horner's syndrome following surgery despite minimal manipulation of sympathetic nerve structures. These clinical signs are usually transient, resolving within 30 days.

All cats suspected of having inflammatory nasopharyngeal polyp should have oral and otic examinations before surgery to determine the extent of the disease process.

Plate 34

Approach to the Ventral Tympanic Bulla: Feline *continued*

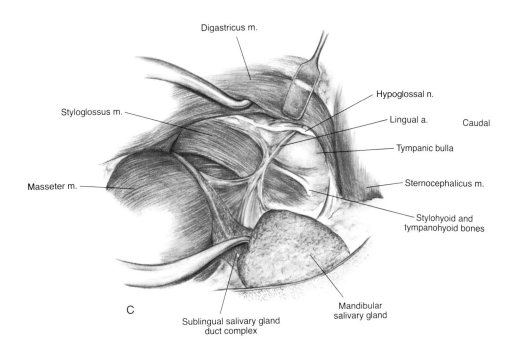

Digastricus m.

Hypoglossal n.

Styloglossus m.

Lingual a.

Caudal

Tympanic bulla

Masseter m.

Sternocephalicus m.

Stylohyoid and
tympanohyoid bones

C

Sublingual salivary gland
duct complex

Mandibular
salivary gland

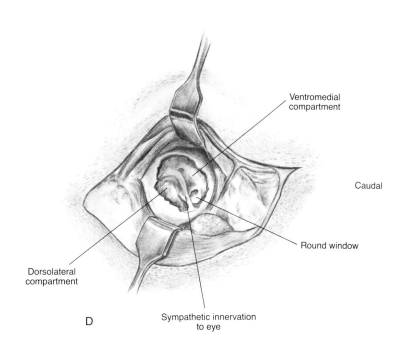

Ventromedial
compartment

Caudal

Round window

Dorsolateral
compartment

D

Sympathetic innervation
to eye

Approach to the Cervical Trachea

INDICATIONS

Tracheotomy for tracheostomy tube placement or foreign body removal, resection and reconstruction for stenosis or neoplasm, permanent tracheostomy, and exploratory surgery for tracheal collapse or trauma.

DESCRIPTION OF THE PROCEDURE

A. The left ventrolateral view of the cervical trachea shows anatomic structures that may require consideration during surgery of the trachea. These structures include the esophagus, the recurrent laryngeal nerve, the thyroid gland, the caudal thyroid artery and vein, the vagosympathetic trunk, the internal carotid artery, and the internal jugular vein.

Plate 35
Approach to the Cervical Trachea

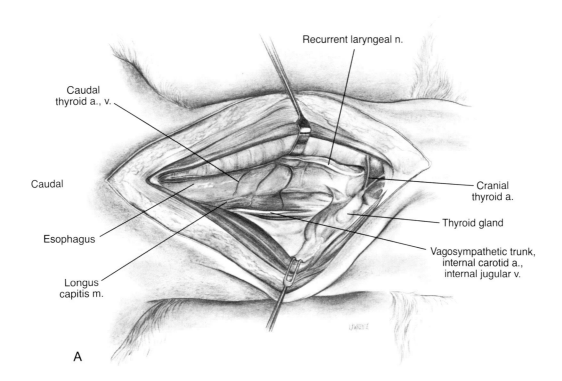

Recurrent laryngeal n.

Caudal
thyroid a., v.

Caudal

Esophagus

Longus
capitis m.

Cranial
thyroid a.

Thyroid gland

Vagosympathetic trunk,
internal carotid a.,
internal jugular v.

A

Approach to the Cervical Trachea *continued*

DESCRIPTION OF THE PROCEDURE *continued*

B. The patient is positioned in dorsal recumbency. A ventral midline skin incision is made between the palpable landmarks of the cricoid cartilage of the larynx and the manubrium. Skin incision for tracheostomy tube placement is similar but ends at the cranial third of the trachea.

C. Following incision of the platysma muscle and the subcutaneous tissues, the paired sternohyoideus muscles are divided along the midline. Caudal extension of the incision requires division of the sternocephalicus muscles. The sternohyoideus and sternothyroideus muscles are retracted to expose the trachea. Ligation and division or electrocoagulation of one or more of the the caudal thyroid veins completes the approach.

D. Transverse tracheotomy for tracheostomy tube placement is performed by a horizontal incision of the annular ligament between the third and fourth or fourth and fifth tracheal rings.

CLOSURE

The sternohyoideus muscles are apposed using synthetic absorbable suture in a simple continuous pattern. Subcutaneous tissues are apposed similarly followed by skin apposition using nonabsorbable suture in alternating simple interrupted and vertical mattress patterns.

COMMENTS

Transverse tracheotomy incisions should extend less than half the diameter of the trachea to prevent tracheal disruption at the tracheotomy site. The diameter of the tracheostomy tube should be no greater than half the diameter of the trachea.

Invasive neoplasms and traumatic injuries may disrupt anatomic structures near the trachea (see Fig. **A**), necessitating careful dissection during exploratory or resective procedures.

The tendency of ventral neck skin to invert during wound closure may be prevented by alternating simple interrupted and vertical mattress skin sutures.

Based on a procedure of Munson TO: Injuries of the laryngeal and tracheal cartilages. In Mayer K, LaCroix JV, and Hoskins HP (eds): Canine Surgery. Santa Barbara, CA, American Veterinary Publications, 1957, p 284.

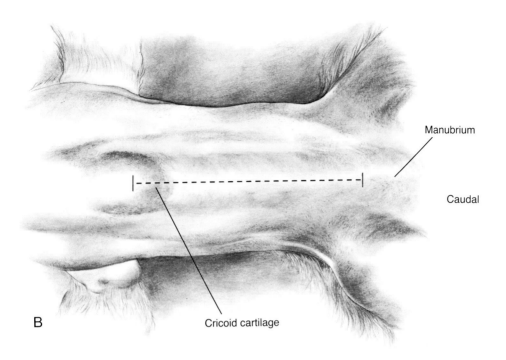

B

Manubrium

Caudal

Cricoid cartilage

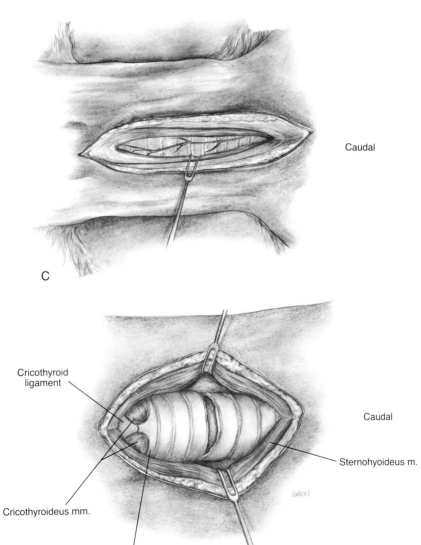

C

Caudal

Cricothyroid
ligament

Caudal

Sternohyoideus m.

Cricothyroideus mm.

Cricoid cartilage

D

121

Thoracic Surgery

- Approach to the Left Thorax by Fourth Intercostal Space Thoracotomy

- Approach to the Left Thorax by Rib Pivot Thoracotomy

- Approach to the Right Thorax by Fifth Intercostal Space Thoracotomy

- Approach to the Right Caudal Thorax by Ninth Intercostal Space Thoracotomy

- Approach to the Ventral Thorax by Median Sternotomy

- Approach to the Thoracic Inlet

- Approach to the Caudal Thorax by Transdiaphragmatic Thoracotomy: Feline

- Intrathoracic Approach to the Left Cranial Esophagus and the Mediastinal Lymph Nodes

- Intrathoracic Approach to the Thymus

- Intrathoracic Approach to the Left Heart Base

- Intrathoracic Approach to the Right Cranial Esophagus, the Trachea, and the Mediastinal Lymph Nodes

- Intrathoracic Approach to the Pericardium and the Right Auricle

- Intrathoracic Approach to the Tracheal Bifurcation and the Tracheobronchial Lymph Nodes

- Intrathoracic Approach to the Hilus of the Right Lung

- Intrathoracic Approach to the Right Caudal Esophagus and the Thoracic Duct

Approach to the Left Thorax by Fourth Intercostal Space Thoracotomy

INDICATIONS

Thoracotomy for limited exploration of the thorax and surgical procedures of left pulmonary, cardiac, and pericardiac structures.

DESCRIPTION OF THE PROCEDURE

A. The patient is positioned in right lateral recumbency over an elevated, padded area (e.g., a rolled towel) placed at the thorax perpendicular to the long axis of the body. A vertical skin incision is made over the fourth intercostal space from the angle of the rib to the costochondral junction.

B. Subcutaneous tissue and the cutaneous trunci muscle are incised to expose the latissimus dorsi muscle and the lateral thoracic nerve.

C. The latissimus dorsi muscle and the lateral thoracic nerve are incised. The thoracotomy is continued by incision of the scalenus muscle ventrally and by separation of the serratus ventralis muscle fibers dorsally.

Plate 36

Approach to the Left Thorax by Fourth Intercostal Space Thoracotomy

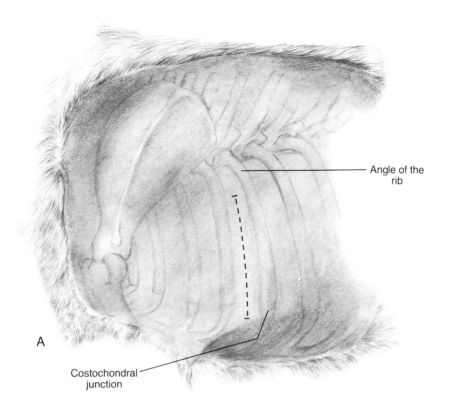

Angle of the rib

Costochondral junction

A

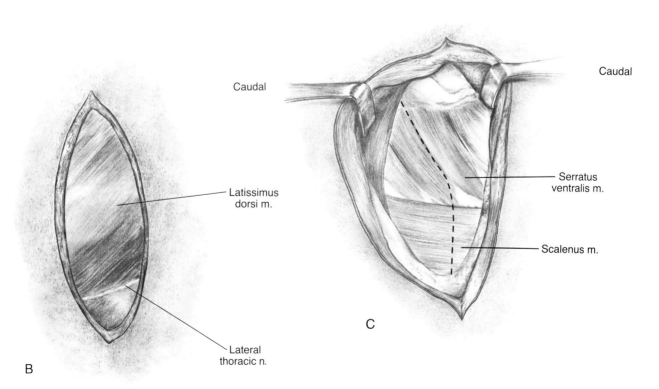

Caudal

Latissimus dorsi m.

Lateral thoracic n.

B

Caudal

Serratus ventralis m.

Scalenus m.

C

Approach to the Left Thorax by Fourth Intercostal Space Thoracotomy *continued*

DESCRIPTION OF THE PROCEDURE *continued*

D. Thoracotomy is completed by division of the external and internal intercostal muscles and of the parietal pleura cranial to the fifth rib, avoiding the intercostal artery, vein, and nerve that course caudal to the fourth rib. The intercostal incision may extend to the tubercle of the rib dorsally and past the costochondral junction ventrally.

CLOSURE

A thoracostomy tube is placed to allow restoration of negative thoracic pressure and fluid removal following wound closure. The rolled towel is removed, and interrupted circumcostal sutures of synthetic absorbable material are preplaced, with the intercostal blood supply caudal to each rib avoided. Care is taken to avoid needle trauma to the inflated lung during suture placement. The sutures are tied to appose the ribs without excessive tension, which may cause rib overlap. Divided and incised muscles are apposed using synthetic absorbable suture in a simple interrupted pattern. Subcutaneous tissues are apposed using similar suture in a simple continuous pattern. Skin is apposed using synthetic nonabsorbable suture in a simple interrupted pattern.

COMMENTS

Extension of the intercostal incision ventral to the costochondral junction should be performed cautiously to avoid the internal thoracic artery and vein coursing adjacent to the sternal ends of the costal cartilages.

The ventral aspect of the latissimus dorsi may be retracted dorsally to avoid myotomy; however, the authors prefer incision because it allows greater exposure.

Intercostal nerve block with long-acting local anesthetic may be administered prior to thoracotomy closure to decrease postoperative pain.

Based on a procedure of Heuer GF, and Dunn GR: Experimental pneumonectomy. Bull Johns Hopkins Hosp 31:31–42, 1920.

Plate 36

Approach to the Left Thorax by Fourth Intercostal Space Thoracotomy *continued*

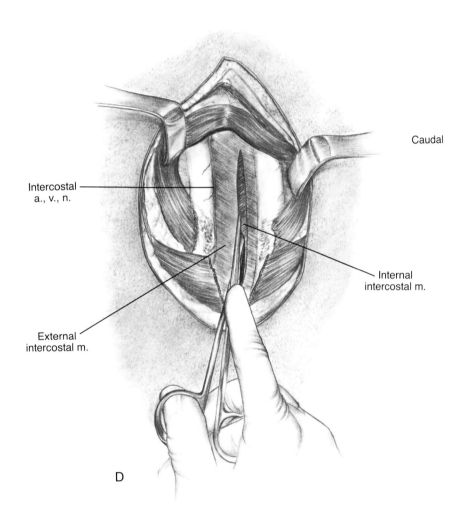

Caudal

Intercostal
a., v., n.

Internal
intercostal m.

External
intercostal m.

D

Approach to the Left Thorax by Rib Pivot Thoracotomy

INDICATIONS

Extended thoracotomy for exploration of the thorax and surgical procedures of left pulmonary, cardiac, and pericardiac structures.

DESCRIPTION OF THE PROCEDURE

A. Following left fourth intercostal space thoracotomy (see p 124), greater exposure of the thoracic structures may be obtained by osteotomy of the adjacent caudal ribs. The previously incised scalenus muscle is elevated and retracted to expose the costochondral junctions of the adjacent caudal ribs.

B. The external and internal intercostal muscles and the costal pleura are incised between the ribs. Osteotomy is performed at the costochondral junction of the fifth and sixth ribs using a bone-cutting instrument. The intercostal artery and vein are ligated following rib osteotomy.

CLOSURE

Costochondral osteotomy is repaired by application of cruciate mattress sutures in the periosteum and the costal cartilage with absorbable or nonabsorbable suture or by hemicerclage with orthopedic wire. The intercostal musculature is apposed using synthetic absorbable suture in a simple interrupted pattern. The thoracotomy is closed as described in Approach to the Left Thorax by Fourth Intercostal Space Thoracotomy (see p 126).

COMMENTS

Rib pivot thoracotomy allows access to the pleural space with large instruments (e.g., stapling devices), assists in the management of unexpected intraoperative complications requiring greater exposure, and facilitates manipulations required to exteriorize large neoplasms.

This procedure can be used to extend any intercostal thoracotomy.

Intercostal nerve block with a long-acting local anesthetic may be administered prior to thoracotomy closure to decrease postoperative pain.

Based on a procedure of Schulman AJ, and Lippincott CL: Rib pivot thoracotomy. Compend Contin Educ Pract Vet 10:927–930, 1988.

Plate 37

Approach to the Left Thorax by Rib Pivot Thoractomy

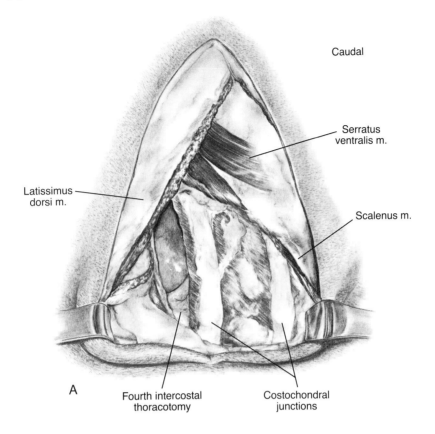

Caudal

Serratus
ventralis m.

Latissimus
dorsi m.

Scalenus m.

A

Fourth intercostal
thoracotomy

Costochondral
junctions

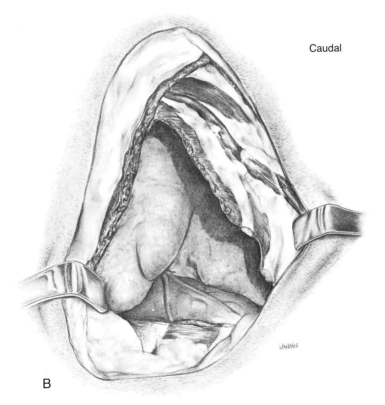

Caudal

B

Approach to the Right Thorax by Fifth Intercostal Space Thoracotomy

INDICATIONS

Thoracotomy for limited exploration of the thorax and surgical procedures of right pulmonary, cardiac, and pericardiac structures.

DESCRIPTION OF THE PROCEDURE

A. The patient is positioned in left lateral recumbency over an elevated, padded area (e.g., a rolled towel) placed at the thorax perpendicular to the long axis of the body. A vertical skin incision is made over the fifth intercostal space from the angle of the rib to the costochondral junction. Subcutaneous tissue and the cutaneous trunci muscle are incised to expose the latissimus dorsi muscle.

B. The latissimus dorsi muscle is incised. Landmarks indicating the proper intercostal space include the dorsal, superficial component of the scalenus muscle, which arises from the fifth rib; serrations of the serratus ventralis muscle; and the origin of the external abdominal oblique muscle from the fifth rib.

Plate 38

Approach to the Right Thorax by Fifth Intercostal Space Thoracotomy

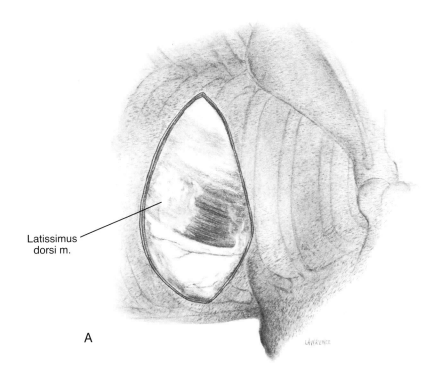

Latissimus
dorsi m.

A

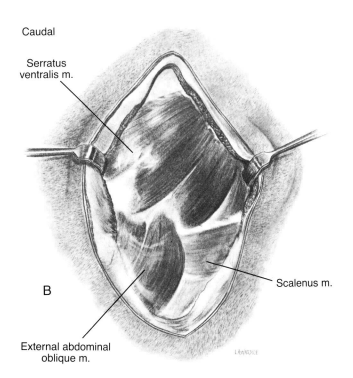

Caudal

Serratus
ventralis m.

Scalenus m.

B

External abdominal
oblique m.

Approach to the Right Thorax by Fifth Intercostal Space Thoracotomy *continued*

DESCRIPTION OF THE PROCEDURE *continued*

C. The thoracotomy is continued by division of the fascial attachment between the scalenus and external abdominal oblique muscles. Elevation of the external abdominal oblique muscle from the fifth rib and division of the serratus ventralis muscle fibers dorsally expose the intercostal musculature. Thoracotomy is completed by division of the external and internal intercostal muscles and of the parietal pleura cranial to the sixth rib, avoiding the intercostal artery, vein, and nerve that course caudal to the fifth rib. The intercostal incision may extend to the tubercle of the rib dorsally and past the costochondral junction ventrally.

CLOSURE

A thoracostomy tube is placed to allow restoration of negative thoracic pressure and removal of fluid following wound closure. The rolled towel is removed, and interrupted circumcostal sutures of synthetic absorbable material are preplaced, with the intercostal blood supply caudal to each rib avoided. Care is taken to avoid needle trauma to the inflated lung during suture placement. The sutures are tied to appose the ribs without excessive tension, which may cause rib overlap. Divided and incised muscles are apposed using synthetic absorbable suture in a simple interrupted pattern. Subcutaneous tissues are apposed using similar suture in a simple continuous pattern. Skin is apposed using synthetic, nonabsorbable suture in a simple interrupted pattern.

COMMENTS

Extension of the intercostal incision ventral to the costochondral junction should be performed cautiously to avoid the internal thoracic artery and vein coursing adjacent to the sternal ends of the costal cartilages.

The ventral aspect of the latissimus dorsi may be retracted dorsally to avoid myotomy; however, the authors prefer incision because it allows greater exposure.

Intercostal nerve block with long-acting local anesthetic may be administered prior to thoracotomy closure to decrease postoperative pain.

Based on a procedure of Heuer GF, and Dunn GR: Experimental pneumonectomy. Bull Johns Hopkins Hosp 31:31–42, 1920.

Plate 38

Approach to the Right Thorax by Fifth Intercostal Space Thoracotomy *continued*

Caudal

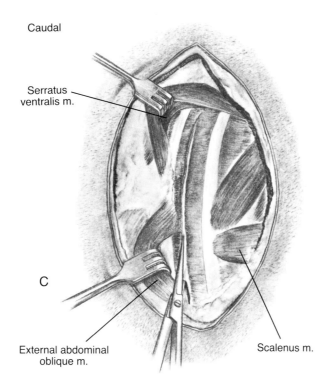

Serratus
ventralis m.

C

External abdominal
oblique m.

Scalenus m.

Approach to the Right Caudal Thorax by Ninth Intercostal Space Thoracotomy

INDICATIONS

Thoracotomy for procedures involving the caudal thoracic vena cava, the esophagus, the right diaphragm, and the thoracic duct.

DESCRIPTION OF THE PROCEDURE

A. The patient is positioned in left lateral recumbency over an elevated, padded area (e.g., a rolled towel) placed at the thorax perpendicular to the long axis of the body. A vertical skin incision is made over the ninth intercostal space from the angle of the rib to the costochondral junction. Subcutaneous tissue and the cutaneous trunci muscle are incised to expose the latissimus dorsi muscle.

B. The latissimus dorsi muscle is incised. Landmarks indicating the proper intercostal space include the caudal aspect of the cranial serratus dorsalis muscle, which has points of insertion on the ninth and tenth ribs, and the external abdominal oblique muscle ventrally. Thoracotomy is completed by division of the external and internal intercostal muscles and of the parietal pleura cranial to the tenth rib, avoiding the intercostal artery, vein, and nerve that course caudal to the ninth rib.

CLOSURE

A thoracostomy tube is placed to allow restoration of negative thoracic pressure and fluid removal following wound closure. The rolled towel is removed, and interrupted circumcostal sutures of synthetic absorbable material are preplaced, with the intercostal blood supply caudal to each rib avoided. Care is taken to avoid needle trauma to the inflated lung during suture placement. The sutures are tied to appose the ribs without excessive tension, which may cause rib overlap. Divided and incised muscles are apposed using synthetic absorbable suture in a simple interrupted pattern. Subcutaneous tissues are apposed using similar suture in a simple continuous pattern. Skin is apposed using synthetic nonabsorbable suture in a simple interrupted pattern.

COMMENTS

Extension of the intercostal incision ventral to the costochondral junction should be performed cautiously to avoid the internal thoracic artery and vein coursing adjacent to the sternal ends of the costal cartilages.

Intercostal nerve block with long-acting local anesthetic may be administered prior to thoracotomy closure to decrease postoperative pain.

Based on a procedure of Patterson DF, and Munson TO: Traumatic chylothorax in small animals treated by ligation of the thoracic duct. J Am Vet Med Assoc 133:452–458, 1958.

Plate 39

Approach to the Right Caudal Thorax by Ninth Intercostal Space Thoractomy

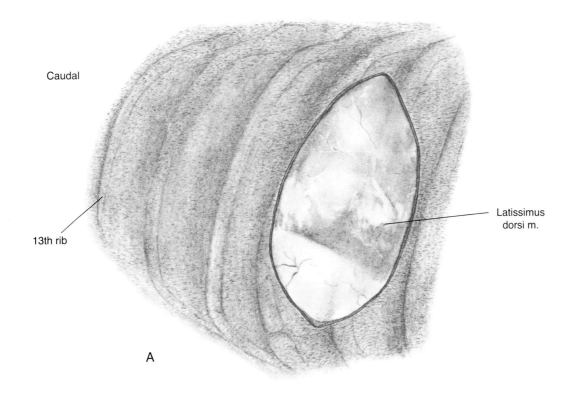

Caudal

13th rib

Latissimus
dorsi m.

A

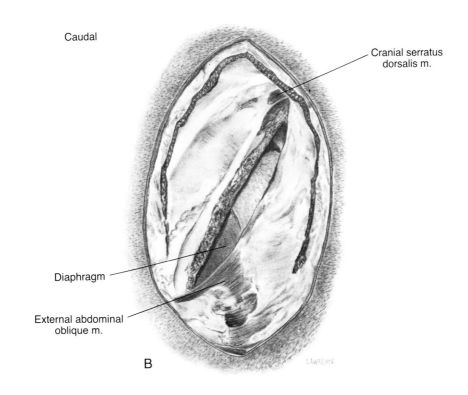

Caudal

Cranial serratus
dorsalis m.

Diaphragm

External abdominal
oblique m.

B

Approach to the Ventral Thorax by Median Sternotomy

INDICATIONS

Thoracotomy for procedures involving the ventral thorax and for exploration of the entire thoracic cavity.

DESCRIPTION OF THE PROCEDURE

A. The patient is positioned in dorsal recumbency. A ventral midline skin incision is made over the sternum. The incision may be combined with either an exploratory celiotomy incision or a ventral cervical neck incision if necessary.

B. Subcutaneous tissues are incised to expose the origin of the superficial and deep pectoralis muscles on the sternebrae.

C. Pectoral musculature is elevated from the ventral sternebrae with a sharp periosteal elevator to provide exposure for sternebrae osteotomy using an oscillating bone saw or an osteotome and a mallet. During muscle elevation, hemostatic methods may be required for the multiple ventral cutaneous branches of the internal thoracic artery and vein. Osteotomy may be extended in a cranial or caudal direction, depending on the goals of the operative procedure. The sternotomy (osteotomy) does not routinely extend through the xiphoid and the manubrium.

CLOSURE

A thoracostomy tube is placed to allow restoration of negative thoracic pressure and fluid removal following wound closure. Multiple techniques have been recommended for maintenance of sternebrae apposition. A figure-eight or cruciate pattern including the costosternal junction using heavy, nonabsorbable suture or orthopedic wire provides a stable sternebrae closure. The superficial and deep pectoralis muscles are apposed using synthetic absorbable suture in a cruciate mattress pattern. Subcutaneous tissues are apposed using similar suture in a simple continuous pattern with periodic tacking to the muscular layer to decrease dead space. Skin is apposed using nonabsorbable suture in a simple interrupted pattern.

COMMENTS

Adequate stabilization of sternebrae minimizes postoperative complications, which may include pain, pneumothorax, and pleurocutaneous air leakage.

Incomplete sternotomy that preserves either the xiphoid cartilage or the manubrium is adequate for most procedures. Preservation of either structure contributes to sternotomy stability following surgery.

Caudal sternotomy may require partial incision of the diaphragm and cranial celiotomy for adequate exposure.

Based on a procedure of Markowitz J, Archibald J, and Downie HG: Experimental surgery of the heart. In *Experimental Surgery, Baltimore, Williams & Wilkins, 1959, p 570.*

Plate 40

Approach to the Ventral Thorax by Median Sternotomy

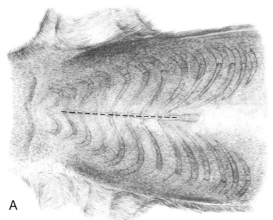

A

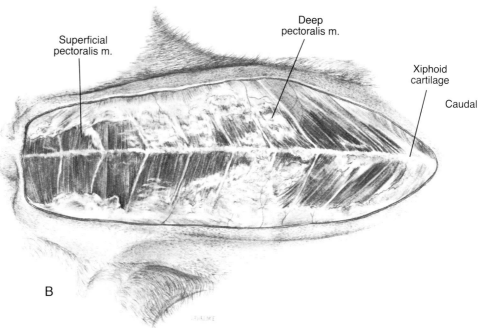

Superficial
pectoralis m.

Deep
pectoralis m.

Xiphoid
cartilage

Caudal

B

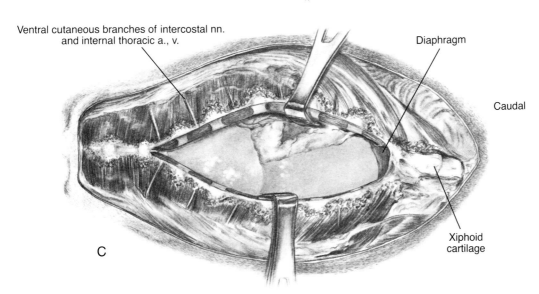

Ventral cutaneous branches of intercostal nn.
and internal thoracic a., v.

Diaphragm

Caudal

Xiphoid
cartilage

C

Approach to the Thoracic Inlet

INDICATIONS

Exploratory surgery of the caudal cervical region and the thoracic inlet for esophageal or tracheal foreign body removal, for repair of perforation, and for application of prosthetic devices for collapsing trachea.

DESCRIPTION OF THE PROCEDURE

A. The patient is positioned in dorsal recumbency. A ventral midline skin incision is made from the cranial trachea to the third sternebra. The sternohyoideus and sternocephalicus muscles are divided on the midline. The subcutaneous tissue ventral to the manubrium is incised to expose the superficial pectoralis muscle.

B. The sternohyoideus and sternocephalicus muscles are lateralized using a self-retaining retractor to allow observation of the esophagus, the trachea, the common carotid artery, and the vagosympathetic trunk.

Plate 41

Approach to the Thoracic Inlet

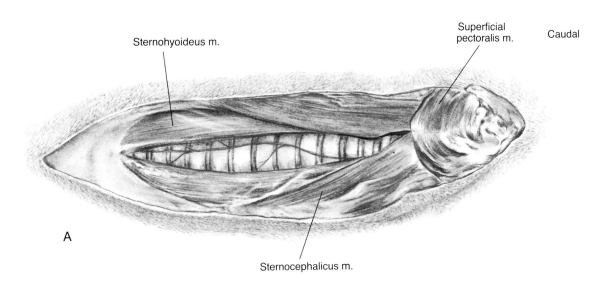

Sternohyoideus m.

Superficial pectoralis m.

Caudal

Sternocephalicus m.

A

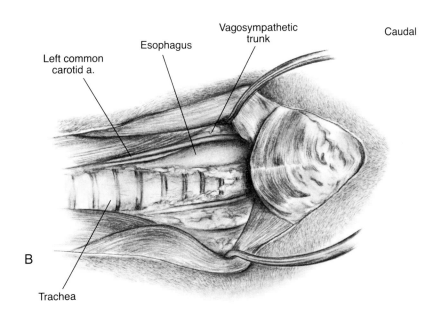

Left common carotid a.

Esophagus

Vagosympathetic trunk

Caudal

Trachea

B

Approach to the Thoracic Inlet *continued*

DESCRIPTION OF THE PROCEDURE *continued*

C. Traction on the superficial pectoralis muscle and the manubrium followed by incision of the mediastinal pleura exposes the thoracic inlet and the cranial mediastinum.

D. The surgical approach may be extended to increase mediastinal exposure by incision of the superficial and deep pectoralis muscles and by osteotomy of cranial sternebrae using an osteotome and a mallet, bone cutters, or an oscillating bone saw. The common carotid arteries form a wishbone shape emanating from the brachycephalic trunk. Major tributaries to the cranial vena cava should be gently retracted to continue the surgical procedure caudally.

CLOSURE

Closure of partial sternotomy is similar to closure used for median sternotomy (p 136). The pectoralis muscles are apposed on the midline using synthetic absorbable suture in a simple interrupted pattern. The sternohyoideus and sternocephalicus muscles are apposed similarly, followed by closure of subcutaneous tissues using synthetic absorbable suture in a simple continuous pattern. The skin is apposed using synthetic nonabsorbable suture in a simple interrupted pattern.

COMMENTS

If thoracotomy is performed, a thoracostomy tube should be placed to allow restoration of negative thoracic pressure and fluid removal following wound closure.

Surgery limited to the caudal cervical area should be performed with the knowledge that the cranial thorax is easily entered inadvertently, requiring the surgeon to administer positive-pressure ventilation.

Meticulous apposition of muscle layers in the caudal cervical area will minimize the risks of postoperative pneumothorax and subcutaneous emphysema related to pleuro-cutaneous air leakage.

Plate 41

Approach to the Thoracic Inlet *continued*

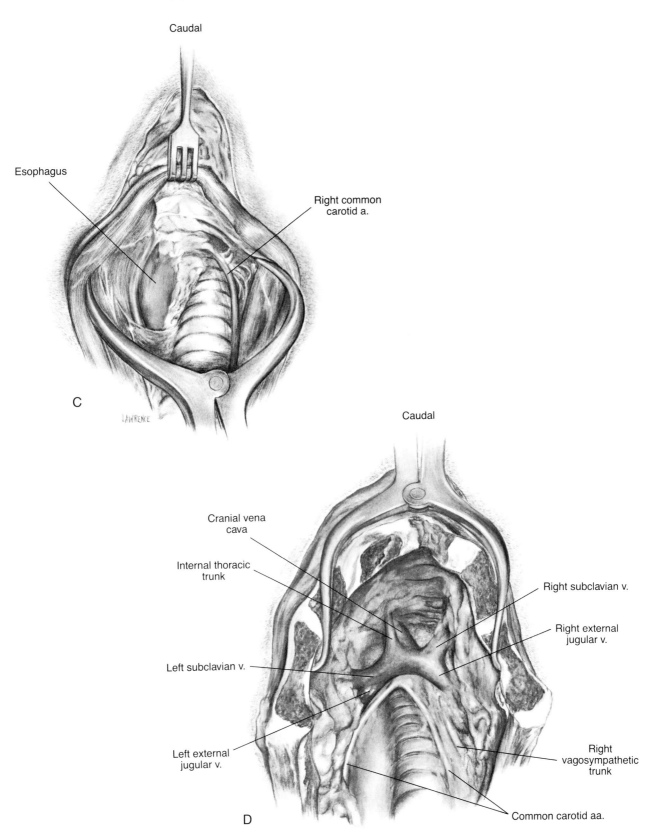

Caudal

Esophagus

Right common
carotid a.

C

LAWRENCE

Caudal

Cranial vena
cava

Internal thoracic
trunk

Right subclavian v.

Right external
jugular v.

Left subclavian v.

Left external
jugular v.

Right
vagosympathetic
trunk

Common carotid aa.

D

Approach to the Caudal Thorax by Transdiaphragmatic Thoracotomy: Feline

INDICATIONS

Thoracotomy following cranial celiotomy for thoracic duct exploration and ligation as a component of management of chylothorax.

DESCRIPTION OF THE PROCEDURE

A. The patient is positioned in dorsal recumbency. An approach to the cranial abdomen is performed as described on p 166. Moistened laparotomy pads are used to protect the abdominal wall, followed by placement of a self-retaining abdominal retractor. Moistened laparotomy pads are placed over abdominal viscera, and a malleable ribbon retractor is used to retract structures of the left cranial quadrant of the abdomen. The diaphragm is incised from a location 2 cm dorsolateral to the xiphoid cartilage dorsally toward the left diaphragmatic crus until adequate exposure of the caudal thoracic aorta is achieved. Stay sutures are placed in the diaphragm to minimize the risk of trauma associated with retraction.

B. Vital dye injected into an accessible abdominal lymph node aids visualization of the thoracic duct coursing along the left dorsal aspect of the thoracic aorta. The caudal mediastinal pleura is incised. Retraction of the aorta ventrally and to the right may facilitate thoracic duct manipulation. The thoracic duct is divided following occlusion with silk suture ligatures or hemostatic clips.

CLOSURE

The diaphragm is apposed using synthetic nonabsorbable or absorbable suture in a simple or interlocking continuous pattern. A thoracostomy tube should be placed to allow restoration of negative thoracic pressure and removal of residual chylous fluid following wound closure. The celiotomy is closed as described in Approach to the Cranial Abdomen (p 168).

COMMENTS

This approach provides easy access to the abdomen for exploratory surgery and lymph node injection with vital dye. However, only limited exploration of the thorax is possible.

There may be multiple branches of the thoracic duct emanating from the cisterna chyli requiring ligation.

The left vagus nerve courses near the thoracic duct and should be avoided.

In the dog, the thoracic duct courses along the right dorsal aspect of the aorta. An approach similar to that for the cat followed by manipulation of the aorta provides access to the thoracic duct in the dog.

Based on a procedure of Martin RA, Richards DLS, Barber DL, et al: Transdiaphragmatic approach to thoracic duct ligation in the cat. Vet Surg 17:22–26, 1988.

Plate 42

Approach to the Caudal Thorax by Transdiaphragmatic Thoracotomy: Feline

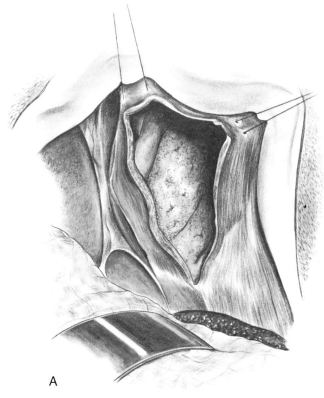

A

Caudal

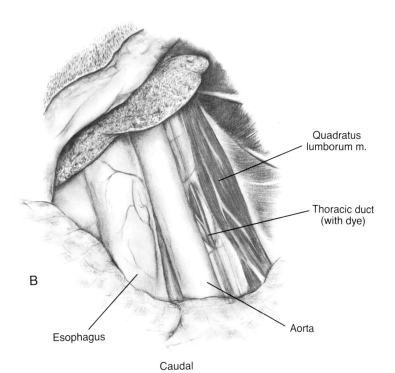

B

Quadratus lumborum m.

Thoracic duct (with dye)

Esophagus

Aorta

Caudal

Intrathoracic Approach to the Left Cranial Esophagus and the Mediastinal Lymph Nodes

INDICATIONS

Cranial esophagotomy for foreign body removal or partial esophagectomy for neoplasia, and lymph node biopsy for clinical staging of thoracic neoplasms.

DESCRIPTION OF THE PROCEDURE

A. Following left third intercostal space thoracotomy, which is performed similar to fourth intercostal space thoracotomy (see p 124), a rib retractor is positioned to expose structures of the left cranial thorax. The left cranial lung lobe is packed off caudally to allow visualization of structures of the left cranial mediastinum.

Plate 43

Intrathoracic Approach to the Left Cranial Esophagus and the Mediastinal Lymph Nodes

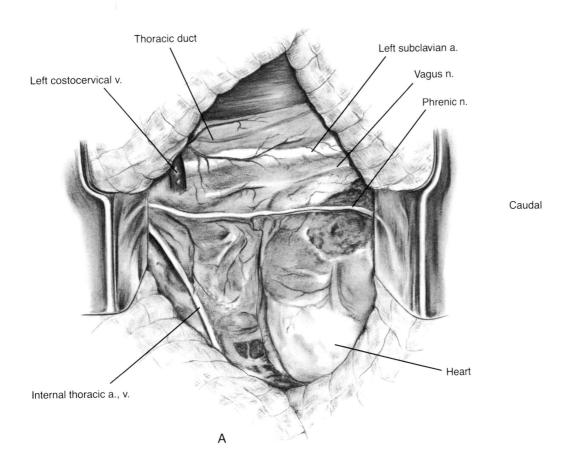

Thoracic duct

Left costocervical v.

Left subclavian a.

Vagus n.

Phrenic n.

Caudal

Internal thoracic a., v.

Heart

A

Intrathoracic Approach to the Left Cranial Esophagus and the Mediastinal Lymph Nodes *continued*

DESCRIPTION OF THE PROCEDURE *continued*

B. The cranial mediastinal pleura is incised dorsal to the left subclavian artery. A vein retractor may be used to provide ventral retraction of the pleura, the left subclavian artery, and the vagus nerve, exposing the esophagus and the trachea.

C. For biopsy of mediastinal lymph nodes, the cranial mediastinal pleura is incised between the phrenic and vagus nerves. A small incision is made ventral to the phrenic nerve, and moistened umbilical tape is used to provide ventral retraction of the phrenic nerve. The location and the number of the cranial mediastinal lymph nodes may vary; however, the mediastinal lymph node ventral to the brachycephalic trunk is consistent.

CLOSURE

Pleural incisions are not sutured. Esophagotomy or esophageal anastomosis is sutured in two layers including the mucosa and submucosa, and the muscular layer. Synthetic nonabsorbable or absorbable suture may be used in simple interrupted patterns. Closure of the thoracotomy is similar to closure described in Approach to the Left Thorax by Fourth Intercostal Space Thoracotomy (see p 126).

COMMENTS

Suppurative mediastinitis may be life-threatening. Thorough packing-off of the operative field for invasive surgery involving the esophagus will decrease contamination of the mediastinum.

Digital occlusion of the esophagus cranial and caudal to the esophageal suture line followed by instillation of sterile saline using a syringe and a 22-gauge needle will allow detection of leaks, which may be repaired with additional simple interrupted sutures.

The most frequently recommended approach to the cranial esophagus is by right cranial thoracotomy, because it avoids major vessels. However, the authors prefer approach by left cranial thoracotomy because it obviates tracheal manipulation and allows major vessels of the left cranial mediastinum to be readily observed and avoided.

Plate 43

Intrathoracic Approach to the Left Cranial Esophagus and the Mediastinal Lymph Nodes *continued*

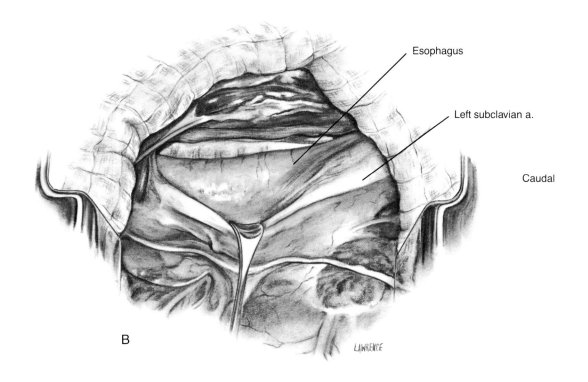

Esophagus

Left subclavian a.

Caudal

B

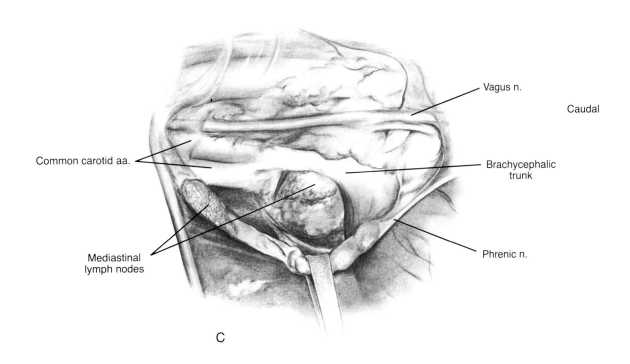

Vagus n.

Caudal

Common carotid aa.

Brachycephalic trunk

Mediastinal lymph nodes

Phrenic n.

C

Intrathoracic Approach to the Thymus

INDICATIONS

Thymectomy for neoplasia of the thymus.

DESCRIPTION OF THE PROCEDURE

A. Following left third intercostal space thoracotomy, which is performed similar to fourth intercostal space thoracotomy (see p 124), a rib retractor is positioned to expose structures of the left cranial thorax. The thymoma is located cranial to the heart and may extend to the right cranial chest. The mass is separated from adjacent pericardial and pleural surfaces by sharp and blunt dissection. The location of the phrenic and vagus nerves should be noted.

B. The left internal thoracic artery and its branch, the pericardiacophrenic artery, are usually engulfed by the mass, requiring ligation of the internal thoracic artery on the dorsal and ventral aspects of the mass. For the same reason, the internal thoracic vein requires ligation in similar locations.

Visualization of the internal thoracic vein as it enters the cranial vena cava is accomplished by sharp dissection ventral to the phrenic nerve. In 50% of canine patients, the internal thoracic vein is unpaired as it enters the cranial vena cava. In the other 50%, the vein is paired with the right entering the cranial vena cava and the left entering the brachicephalic vein.

C. The mass is displaced dorsally to allow visualization and ligation of the internal thoracic artery and vein. Excisional biopsy should be performed on the sternal lymph node to aid staging of the thymic neoplasm.

CLOSURE

Closure of the thoracotomy is similar to closure described in Approach to the Left Thorax by Fourth Intercostal Space Thoracotomy (see p 126).

COMMENTS

Thymomas are invasive, friable neoplasms in the dog. The cranial vena cava may be affected, requiring venotomy for tumor removal. Hemostatic clips decrease operative time.

Postoperative chemotherapy should be considered because complete resection is difficult and tumor cells may seed the thoracic cavity.

Plate 44

Intrathoracic Approach to the Thymus

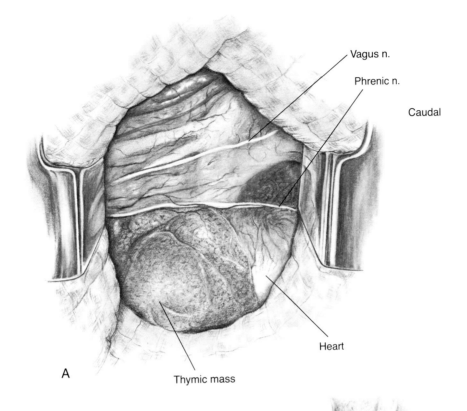

Vagus n.

Phrenic n.

Caudal

Heart

Thymic mass

A

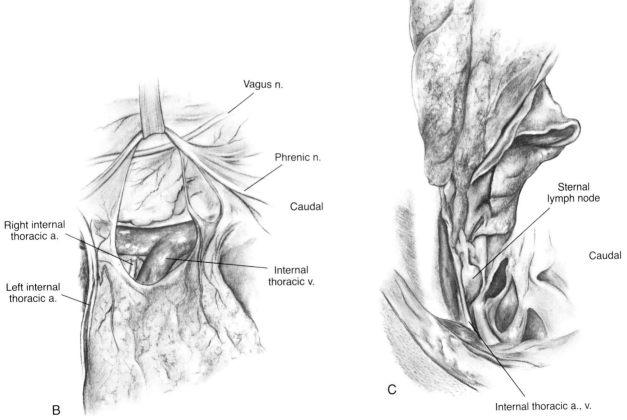

Vagus n.

Phrenic n.

Caudal

Right internal
thoracic a.

Left internal
thoracic a.

Internal
thoracic v.

B

Sternal
lymph node

Caudal

Internal thoracic a., v.

C

Intrathoracic Approach to the Left Heart Base

INDICATIONS

Exploratory surgery for lymph node biopsy, lung lobectomy, and surgical correction of patent ductus arteriosus (PDA) and esophageal compression related to persistent right aortic arch.

DESCRIPTION OF THE PROCEDURE

A. Following left fourth intercostal space thoracotomy (see p 124), a rib retractor is positioned to expose structures of the left middle thorax. The left cranial lung lobe is packed off caudally to expose the left heart base. The aortic arch and the left pulmonary artery are obscured by serous pericardium and fat. The phrenic nerve is visualized as it courses over the left auricle. The vagus nerve is isolated using sharp dissection and umbilical tape. Further dissection reveals the left tracheobronchial lymph node.

B. PDA requires ligation to restore normal cardiovascular hemodynamics. Pericardial tissue is incised longitudinally between the vagus nerve and the phrenic nerve. A small incision is made in the mediastinal pleura dorsal to the vagus nerve, allowing its retraction with umbilical tape. The PDA is apparent between the aortic arch and the pulmonary trunk. A right-angle forcep is used to bluntly dissect along the medial aspect of the ductus. Tearing of the PDA or pulmonary vasculature leading to life-threatening hemorrhage is usually related to excessive tissue trauma medially or inappropriate traction of the ductus.

C. Persistent right aortic arch causes regurgitation related to abnormal compression of the esophagus at the heart base and resultant cranial megaesophagus. The right-sided location of the aortic arch combined with the trachea, pulmonary trunk, and ligamentum arteriosum form a constricting ring around the esophagus at the heart base. Ligation and division of the ligamentum arteriosum relieves the constrictive effect.

CLOSURE

Moistened silk suture is used for PDA and ligamentum arteriosum ligation. Closure of the thoracotomy is similar to closure described in Approach to the Left Thorax by Fourth Intercostal Space Thoracotomy (see p 126).

COMMENTS

A stomach tube placed in the esophagus aids identification of the ligamentum arteriosum and evaluation of esophageal decompression.

Plate 45

Intrathoracic Approach to the Left Heart Base

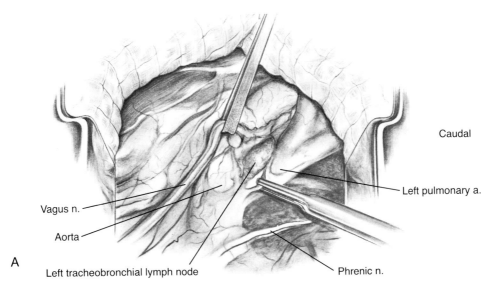

Caudal

Left pulmonary a.

Vagus n.

Aorta

Phrenic n.

Left tracheobronchial lymph node

A

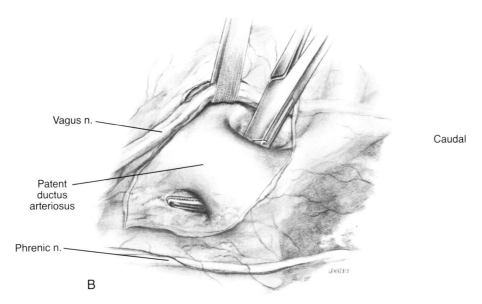

Vagus n.

Caudal

Patent ductus arteriosus

Phrenic n.

B

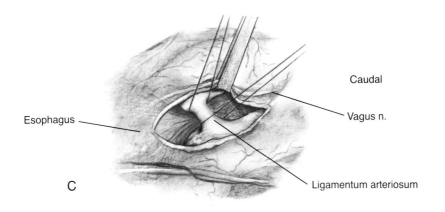

Caudal

Vagus n.

Esophagus

Ligamentum arteriosum

C

Intrathoracic Approach to the Right Cranial Esophagus, the Trachea, and the Mediastinal Lymph Nodes

INDICATIONS

Cranial esophagotomy for foreign body removal or partial esophagectomy for neoplasia, application of prosthetic devices for collapsing trachea, and lymph node biopsy for clinical staging of thoracic neoplasms.

DESCRIPTION OF THE PROCEDURE

A. Following right third intercostal space thoracotomy, which is performed similar to fifth intercostal space thoracotomy (see p 130), a rib retractor is positioned to expose structures of the right cranial thorax. The right cranial lung lobe is packed off to allow visualization of structures of the right cranial mediastinum.

B. The cranial mediastinal pleura is incised dorsal to the right vagus nerve, which courses between the cranial vena cava and the trachea. A small incision is made ventral to the vagus nerve, and moistened umbilical tape is used to provide ventral retraction of the pleura and the vagus nerve. Lateral retraction of the trachea and sharp dissection along the dorsal aspect of the longus colli muscle expose the esophagus.

The location and the number of cranial mediastinal lymph nodes may vary; however, the mediastinal lymph node cranial to the costocervical vein is consistent.

CLOSURE

Pleural incisions are not sutured. Esophagotomy or esophageal anastomosis is sutured in two layers including the mucosa and submucosa, and the muscular layer. Nonabsorbable or absorbable suture with prolonged strength may be used in simple interrupted patterns. Closure of the thoracotomy is similar to closure described in Approach to the Right Thorax by Fifth Intercostal Space Thoracotomy (see p 132).

COMMENTS

Suppurative mediastinitis may be life-threatening. Thorough packing-off of the operative field for invasive surgery involving the esophagus will decrease contamination of the mediastinum.

Digital occlusion of the esophagus cranial and caudal to the esophageal suture line followed by instillation of sterile saline using a syringe and a 22-gauge needle will allow detection of leaks, which may be repaired with additional simple interrupted sutures.

The most frequently recommended approach to the cranial esophagus is by right cranial thoracotomy, because it avoids major vessels. However, the authors prefer approach by left cranial thoracotomy because it obviates tracheal manipulation and allows major vessels of the left cranial mediastinum to be readily observed and avoided.

This is the approach of choice for intrathoracic tracheal surgery.

Plate 46

Intrathoracic Approach to the Right Cranial Esophagus, the Trachea, and the Mediastinal Lymph Nodes

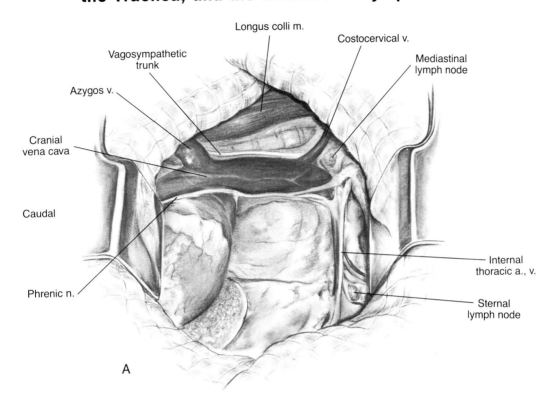

Longus colli m.

Costocervical v.

Vagosympathetic trunk

Mediastinal lymph node

Azygos v.

Cranial vena cava

Caudal

Internal thoracic a., v.

Phrenic n.

Sternal lymph node

A

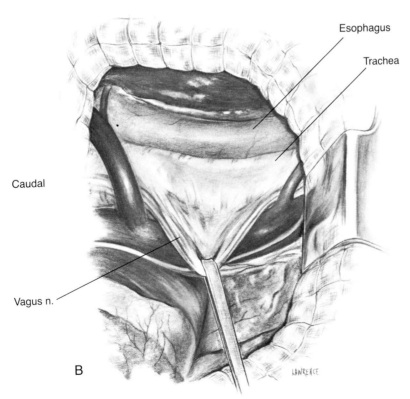

Esophagus

Trachea

Caudal

Vagus n.

B

LAWRENCE

Intrathoracic Approach to the Pericardium and the Right Auricle

INDICATIONS

Pericardectomy for treatment of pericardial effusion in patients with pericarditis refractory to pericardiocenteses, and as a component of surgical management of hemangiosarcoma affecting the right auricle.

DESCRIPTION OF THE PROCEDURE

A. Following right fifth intercostal thoracotomy (see p 130), a rib retractor is positioned to expose structures of the right middle thorax. The right middle and caudal lung lobes are packed off caudally to allow visualization of the right side of the heart and the phrenic nerve. Pericardectomy begins by incision of the pericardium with dissection scissors ventral to the phrenic nerve.

B. Normally small pericardial vessels may become enlarged with pericarditis. Electrosurgery may also be used to perform pericardectomy, provided that the heart is protected by a sterile wooden tongue depressor. Manipulation of the heart by traction on the remaining pericardium assists extension of the pericardial incision cranially and to the left to complete the pericardectomy.

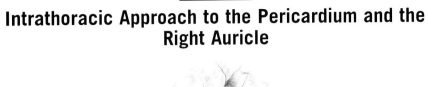

Plate 47
Intrathoracic Approach to the Pericardium and the Right Auricle

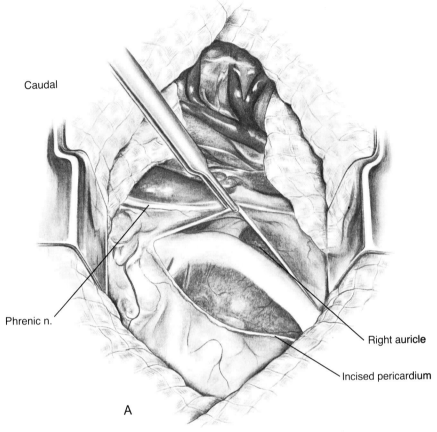

Caudal

Phrenic n.

Right auricle

Incised pericardium

A

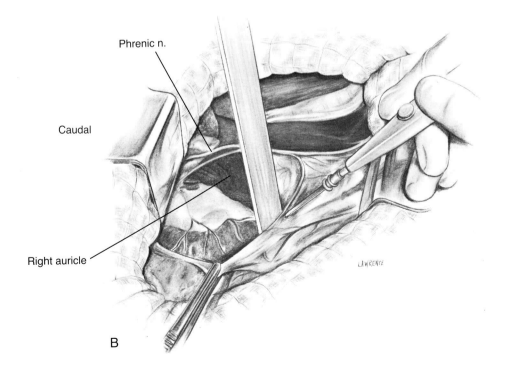

Phrenic n.

Caudal

Right auricle

B

Intrathoracic Approach to the Pericardium and the Right Auricle *continued*

DESCRIPTION OF THE PROCEDURE *continued*

C. The right auricle may be resected for hemangiosarcoma using stapling instrumentation or an atraumatic forcep and suture (inset).

CLOSURE

Resective surgery of the right auricle for neoplasia usually requires a hemostatic mattress suture pattern using nonabsorbable suture proximal to the atraumatic forcep. The auricle is resected distal to the forcep, followed by apposition of the cut auricle surface using similar suture in a simple continuous pattern. The stapling instrument places a double row of hemostatic staples in tissue. The auricle is resected distal to the staple line with dissection scissors. Closure of the thoracotomy is similar to closure described in Approach to the Right Thorax by Fifth Intercostal Space Thoracotomy (see p 132).

COMMENTS

Pericardectomy dorsal to the phrenic nerves is usually not required. A window pericardectomy is usually not sufficient to provide long-term drainage of pericardial effusion to the pleural space.

Median sternotomy provides excellent exposure to both sides of the heart for pericardectomy; however, drainage of pericardial and pleural effusions may complicate healing of the ventral midline sternotomy incision. A disadvantage of lateral thoracotomy is difficulty in performing pericardectomy on the opposite side of the heart.

Long-term prognosis for patients with hemangiosarcoma of the right auricle is poor.

Plate 47

Intrathoracic Approach to the Pericardium and the
Right Auricle *continued*

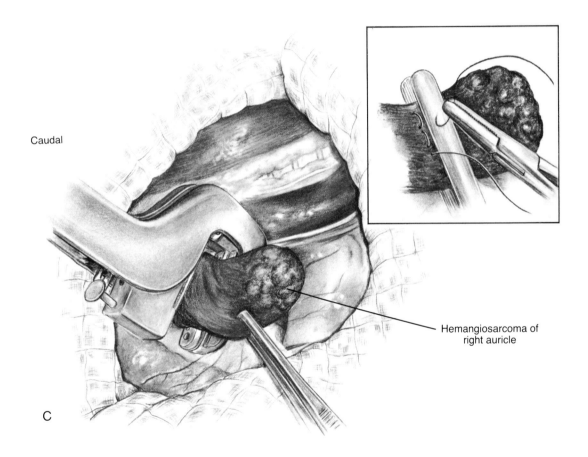

Caudal

Hemangiosarcoma of
right auricle

C

Intrathoracic Approach to the Tracheal Bifurcation and the Tracheobronchial Lymph Nodes

INDICATIONS

Distal tracheotomy for neoplasia or foreign body removal, and lymph node biopsy for clinical staging of thoracic neoplasms.

DESCRIPTION OF THE PROCEDURE

A. Following right fifth intercostal space thoracotomy (see p 130), a rib retractor is positioned to expose structures of the right middle thorax. The right middle and caudal lung lobes are packed off to allow visualization of the azygos vein as it joins the cranial vena cava. The azygos vein may be elevated with umbilical tape to expose the right tracheobronchial lymph node and the vagus nerve.

B. The azygos vein is ligated and divided, and the vagus nerve is isolated and retracted laterally to expose the dorsal tracheal bifurcation and the right and left principal bronchi.

C. The trachealis muscle is incised to allow intraluminal observation of the principal bronchi and the tracheal carina.

CLOSURE

Following foreign body removal, the trachealis muscle may be apposed with synthetic absorbable suture in a simple interrupted pattern. Resective surgery for neoplasia usually requires tracheobronchial reconstruction using similar suture and pattern. Closure of the thoracotomy is similar to closure described in Approach to the Right Thorax by Fifth Intercostal Space Thoracotomy (see p 132).

COMMENTS

Pleural pedicle flaps or an omental pedicle flap brought through the diaphragm may be placed over the sutured site to aid healing and to protect adjacent vascular structures from erosion secondary to rubbing on suture knots.

Plate 48

Intrathoracic Approach to the Tracheal Bifurcation and the Tracheobronchial Lymph Nodes

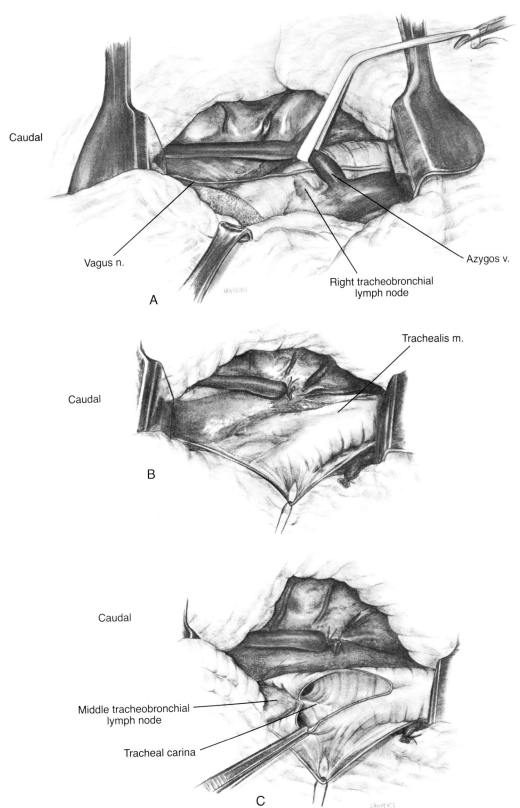

Caudal

Vagus n.

A

Right tracheobronchial
lymph node

Azygos v.

Trachealis m.

Caudal

B

Caudal

Middle tracheobronchial
lymph node

Tracheal carina

C

Intrathoracic Approach to the Hilus of the Right Lung

INDICATIONS

Complete lobectomy for lung cyst, bullae, abscess, torsion, foreign body, and neoplasia.

DESCRIPTION OF THE PROCEDURE

A. Following right fifth intercostal space thoracotomy (see p 130), a rib retractor is positioned to expose structures of the right middle thorax. The right pulmonary artery is isolated ventrolateral to the right bronchi. The right pulmonary vein is isolated ventromedial to the right bronchi. The proximal aspect of each vessel is doubly ligated, beginning with the pulmonary artery to control blood supply to the affected lobe. Dissection of the lung parenchyma may be required to provide a distal location for vessel ligation.

B. The lobar bronchus supplying the caudal and accessory lung lobes is isolated using a curved forcep following sharp dissection.

C. A second clamp is placed in cross-clamp fashion, and the bronchus is resected. The bronchus is sutured proximal to the remaining clamp.

CLOSURE

Pulmonary vessels are ligated with moistened silk suture. The bronchus is sutured with synthetic nonabsorbable suture using preplaced interrupted horizontal mattress sutures or a continuous horizontal mattress pattern. The distal end of the bronchus may be oversewn with similar suture in a simple continuous pattern. Closure of the thoracotomy is similar to closure described in Approach to the Right Thorax by Fifth Intercostal Space Thoracotomy (p 132).

COMMENTS

Warm saline should be placed in the thoracic cavity to cover the bronchial stump so that one can monitor for air leakage during positive-pressure ventilation.

The bronchial closure may be augmented by a pleural pedicle flap to decrease the risk of pneumothorax related to air leakage from the resected bronchus.

Bronchial closure is facilitated by surgical stapling devices.

Plate 49

Intrathoracic Approach to the Hilus of the Right Lung

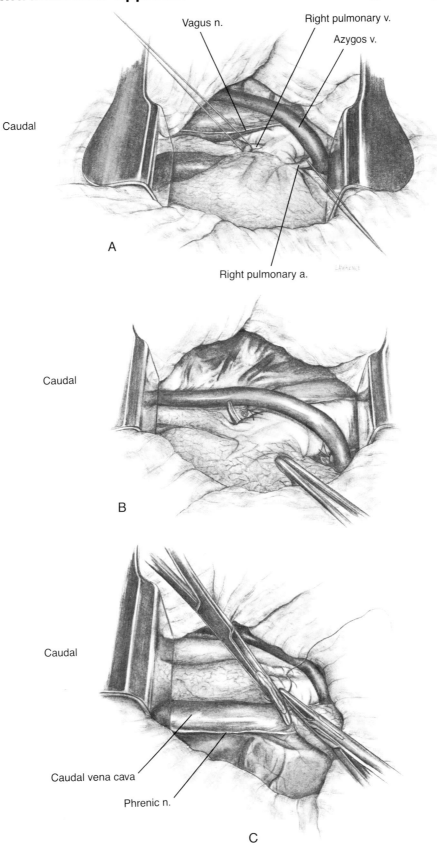

A — Vagus n., Right pulmonary v., Azygos v., Caudal, Right pulmonary a.

B — Caudal

C — Caudal, Caudal vena cava, Phrenic n.

Intrathoracic Approach to the Right Caudal Esophagus and the Thoracic Duct

INDICATIONS

Esophagotomy for neoplasia or foreign body removal and thoracic duct ligation for chylothorax.

DESCRIPTION OF THE PROCEDURE

A. Following ninth intercostal space thoracotomy (see p 134), a rib retractor is positioned to expose structures of the caudal right thorax, including the diaphragm, the right caudal lung lobe, the esophagus, the phrenic nerve, the dorsal branch of the right vagus nerve, the aorta, and the azygos vein with intercostal vein tributaries. The right pulmonary ligament is incised at its junction with the mediastinal pleura. This allows cranial displacement and packing-off of the caudal lung lobe.

B. Atraumatic retraction of the mediastinal pleura, including the dorsal branch of the right vagus nerve, allows visualization of the thoracic duct as it lies in the recessed angle between the aorta ventrally and the azygos vein dorsally. Incision of the mediastinal pleura allows isolation of the thoracic duct.

C. Mobilization of the dorsal and ventral branches of the vagus nerve and isolation of the caudal esophagus are accomplished by sharp and blunt dissection.

CLOSURE

Esophagotomy or esophageal anastomosis is sutured in two layers including the mucosa and submucosa, and the muscular layer using synthetic absorbable suture or monofilament nonabsorbable suture in simple interrupted patterns. Closure of the thoracotomy is similar to closure described in Approach to the Right Thorax by Ninth Intercostal Space Thoracotomy (see p 134).

COMMENTS

Thoracic duct ligation for treatment of chylothorax may be performed using silk suture or stainless steel ligaclips. A vital dye should be injected into a caudal superficial or intraabdominal lymph node prior to exploratory thoracotomy to aid visualization of the thoracic duct. Multiple branches of the thoracic duct may be present.

A transdiaphragmatic approach allows abdominal exploration and vital dye injection followed by thoracic duct ligation, eliminating the need for two operative procedures.

The thoracic duct in the cat courses along the dorsal left aspect of the aorta, requiring left ninth intercostal space thoracotomy for transthoracic ligation.

Plate 50

Intrathoracic Approach to the Right Caudal Esophagus and the Thoracic Duct

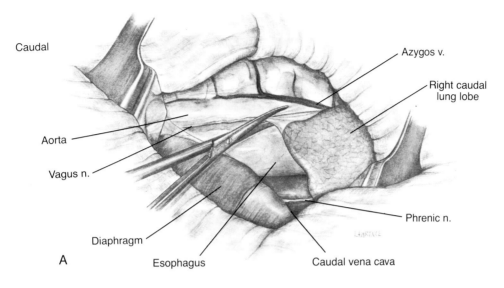

Caudal

Azygos v.

Right caudal
lung lobe

Aorta

Vagus n.

Phrenic n.

Diaphragm

Esophagus

Caudal vena cava

A

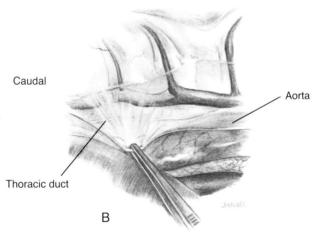

Caudal

Aorta

Thoracic duct

B

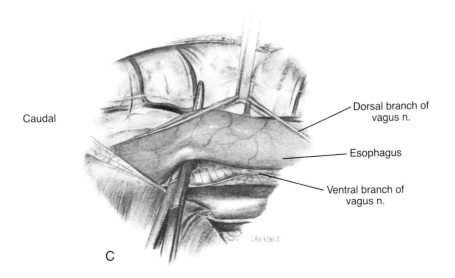

Caudal

Dorsal branch of
vagus n.

Esophagus

Ventral branch of
vagus n.

C

Abdominal Surgery

- Approach to the Abdomen by Cranioventral Midline Celiotomy

- Approach to the Abdomen by Cranioventral-Paracostal Celiotomy

- Approach to the Abdomen by Caudoventral Midline Celiotomy in the Female Dog

- Approach to the Abdomen by Caudoventral Midline Celiotomy in the Male Dog

- Approach to the Abdomen by Paralumbar Celiotomy

- Approach to the Esophageal Hiatus

- Approach to the Stomach

- Approach to the Pylorus

- Approach to the Pancreas

- Approach to the Small Intestine

- Approach to the Colon

- Approach to the Pelvic Canal

- Approach to the Pelvic Canal and the Rectum (Dorsal)

- Approach to the Spleen

- Approach to the Hepatic Veins

- Approach to the Epiploic Foramen

- Approach to the Extrahepatic Biliary System

- Approach to the Adrenal Glands

- **Approach to the Kidneys**

- **Approach to the Extravesicular Ureter**

- **Approach to the Urinary Bladder and the Intravesicular Ureter**

- **Approach to the Uterus and the Ovary**

- **Approach to the Prostate**

- **Approach to the Medial Iliac Lymph Nodes**

Approach to the Abdomen by Cranioventral Midline Celiotomy

INDICATIONS

Exploratory laparotomy for the diagnosis, prognosis, and treatment of disease involving the cranial abdomen.

DESCRIPTION OF THE PROCEDURE

A. The patient is positioned in dorsal recumbency, and the limbs are secured to the operating table. A ventral midline skin incision is made beginning at the xiphoid cartilage cranially and extending caudally to the area of the umbilical scar.

B. Fatty subcutaneous tissues are sharply incised with a scalpel to expose the external fascia of the rectus abdominis muscle. Hemorrhage from small subcutaneous vessels is controlled by electrocautery or ligation.

Plate 51

Approach to the Abdomen by Cranioventral Midline Celiotomy

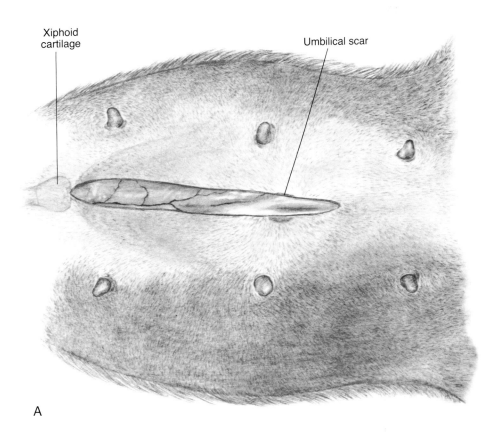

Xiphoid
cartilage

Umbilical scar

A

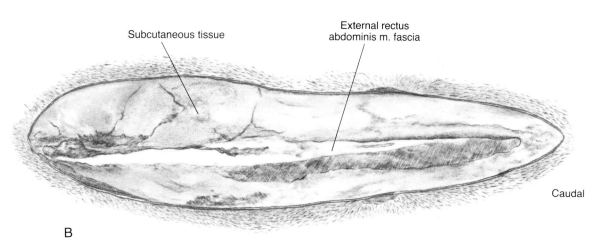

Subcutaneous tissue

External rectus
abdominis m. fascia

Caudal

B

Approach to the Abdomen by Cranioventral Midline Celiotomy *continued*

DESCRIPTION OF THE PROCEDURE *continued*

C. The linea alba is identified, and subcutaneous tissue attachments to the linea alba are incised.

D. The abdominal cavity is entered at the linea alba by tenting the abdominal wall, after which a sharp incision is made with a scalpel. A scalpel or scissors may be used to extend the fascial incision to near the cranial and caudal extent of the skin incision. In the cranial abdomen, visualization of abdominal viscera is obscured by the presence of the falciform ligament attached to the abdominal wall.

E. Exploration and visualization of the abdomen are enhanced by excision of the falciform ligament using scissors or electrocautery. The cranial aspect of the ligament is clamped and ligated to prevent hemorrhage. Laparotomy pads are used to protect the abdominal wall, and self-retaining retractors are placed to assist exposure.

CLOSURE

The abdominal wall is closed with synthetic absorbable suture in a simple interrupted pattern. Subcutaneous tissues are apposed, with care being taken to minimize dead space between the subcutaneous tissue and external rectus abdominis muscle fascia. The skin is closed with nonabsorbable suture in a simple interrupted pattern.

COMMENTS

A generous incision aids exposure of abdominal viscera. The incision should be extended caudally as needed, depending on the operative procedure. Some surgeons prefer to divide the falciform ligament digitally and leave it attached to the abdominal wall.

Closure of the abdominal wall following a midline approach (incision of the linea alba) is accomplished by taking full-thickness bites of the abdominal wall. If the incision is lateral to the linea alba with muscular tissue exposed, the external rectus abdominis muscle fascia is closed without including muscle. The abdominal wall may also be closed with a simple continuous pattern using synthetic nonabsorbable suture.

The authors prefer a continuous intradermal-subcutaneous pattern, which minimizes dead space and gives excellent skin apposition.

Skin sutures should be placed without tension.

Plate 51

Approach to the Abdomen by Cranioventral Midline
Celiotomy *continued*

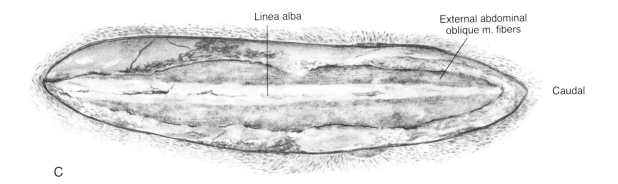

Linea alba

External abdominal oblique m. fibers

Caudal

C

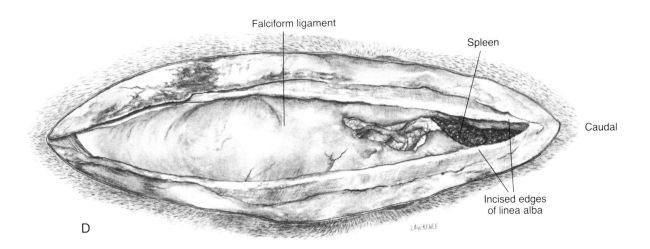

Falciform ligament

Spleen

Caudal

Incised edges of linea alba

D

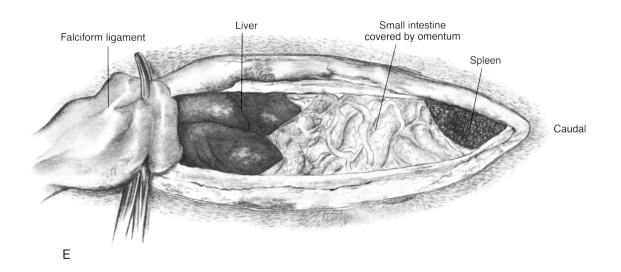

Falciform ligament

Liver

Small intestine covered by omentum

Spleen

Caudal

E

Approach to the Abdomen by Cranioventral-Paracostal Celiotomy

INDICATIONS

Disease involving the right or left cranial abdominal quadrants, in which increased exposure of the cranial abdomen is required.

DESCRIPTION OF THE PROCEDURE

A. The procedure is initiated as described in Approach to the Abdomen by Cranioventral Midline Celiotomy (see p 166). The skin incision is continued laterally from the xiphoid cartilage approximately 1 cm caudal to the last rib.

B. Subcutaneous tissue is sharply incised, after which the fascia of the rectus abdominis muscle and the fibers of the external abdominal oblique, internal abdominal oblique, and transversus abdominis muscles, respectively, are incised.

C. The peninsular abdominal muscle flap that has been created is retracted, exposing the craniolateral abdomen.

CLOSURE

The closure begins by approximation of the abdominal wall at the junction of the combined ventral and paracostal incisions near the xiphoid cartilage. The linea alba is closed with synthetic absorbable suture in a simple interrupted pattern. Each muscle layer of the paracostal incision is closed with a continuous pattern of synthetic absorbable suture. Subcutaneous tissues are apposed with absorbable suture in a continuous or interrupted pattern. The skin is closed with nonabsorbable suture in a simple interrupted pattern.

COMMENTS

This approach will facilitate exposure of the liver, the biliary system, and the diaphragm on the left or right side. Caution should be used when incising the abdominal wall in the area of the xiphoid cartilage. Inadvertent incision of the diaphragm results in pneumothorax.

The linea alba may be closed with a simple continuous pattern using synthetic nonabsorbable suture.

Plate 52
Approach to the Abdomen by Cranioventral-Paracostal Celiotomy

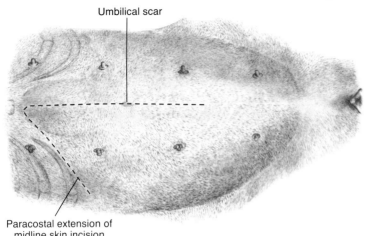

Umbilical scar

Paracostal extension of
midline skin incision

A

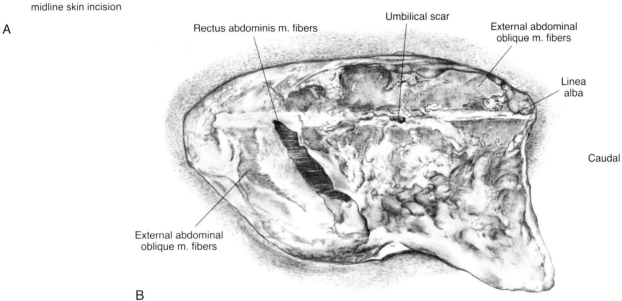

Rectus abdominis m. fibers

Umbilical scar

External abdominal
oblique m. fibers

Linea
alba

Caudal

External abdominal
oblique m. fibers

B

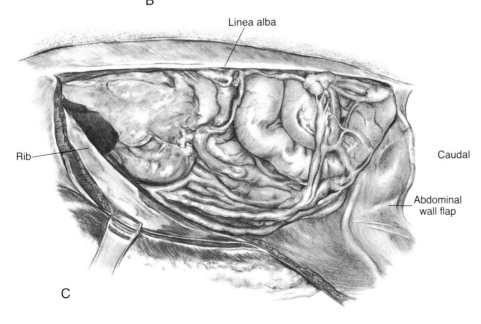

Linea alba

Rib

Caudal

Abdominal
wall flap

C

Approach to the Abdomen by Caudoventral Midline Celiotomy in the Female Dog

INDICATIONS

Exploratory laparotomy for the diagnosis, prognosis, and treatment of disease involving the caudal abdomen.

DESCRIPTION OF THE PROCEDURE

A. The patient is placed in dorsal recumbency, and the limbs are secured to the operating table. A ventral midline skin incision is made beginning at the umbilical scar cranially and extending to the level of the pecten ossis pubis caudally.

B. Subcutaneous tissues are sharply incised to expose the external rectus abdominis muscle fascia and the linea alba.

C. The abdominal cavity is entered by tenting the abdominal wall cranially, after which the linea alba is sharply incised. Extension of the incision is performed using a scalpel or scissors.

CLOSURE

The abdominal wall is closed with synthetic absorbable suture in a simple interrupted pattern. Subcutaneous tissues are apposed with absorbable suture in a continuous or interrupted pattern. The skin is closed with nonabsorbable suture in a simple interrupted pattern.

COMMENTS

The falciform ligament in the caudal half of the abdomen is sparse and does not obscure visualization of the viscera. In the caudal portion of the abdomen, the linea alba becomes thin and when incised tends to retract, exposing muscle fibers of the rectus abdominis muscle. Proper closure technique includes engaging only the external rectus abdominis muscle fascia and not the muscle fibers when closing the caudal aspect of the incision.

Plate 53

Approach to the Abdomen by Caudoventral Midline Celiotomy in the Female Dog

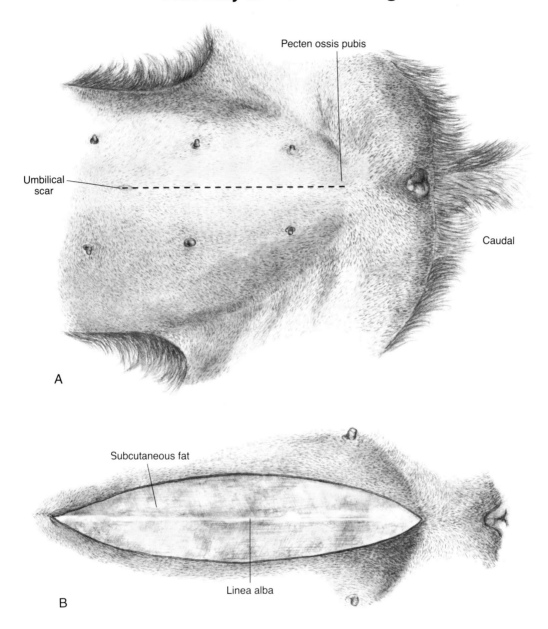

Pecten ossis pubis

Umbilical scar

Caudal

A

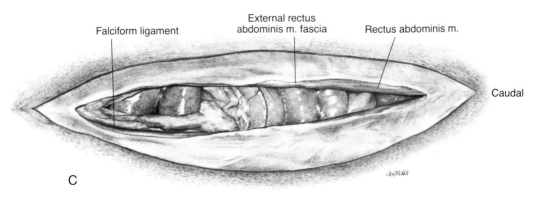

Subcutaneous fat

Linea alba

B

Falciform ligament

External rectus abdominis m. fascia

Rectus abdominis m.

Caudal

C

Approach to the Abdomen by Caudoventral Midline Celiotomy in the Male Dog

INDICATIONS

Exploratory laparotomy for the diagnosis, prognosis, and treatment of disease involving the caudal abdomen.

DESCRIPTION OF THE PROCEDURE

A. The patient is positioned in dorsal recumbency, and the limbs are secured to the operating table. A ventral midline skin incision is made beginning at the umbilical scar cranially; the incision continues caudally and gently curves to the left or right of the penis and prepuce and ends at the level of the pecten ossis pubis caudally.

Plate 54

Approach to the Abdomen by Caudoventral Midline Celiotomy in the Male Dog

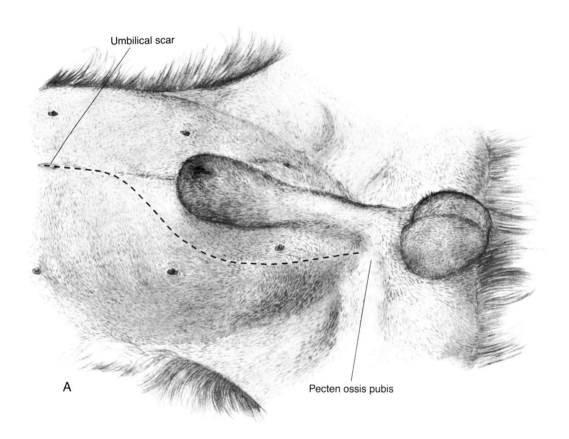

Umbilical scar

Pecten ossis pubis

A

Approach to the Abdomen by Caudoventral Midline Celiotomy in the Male Dog *continued*

DESCRIPTION OF THE PROCEDURE *continued*

B. A towel clamp is used to place the prepuce outside the surgical field. Fibers of the protractor preputii muscle are incised as they course obliquely through the subcutaneous tissue at the cranial aspect of the prepuce. Large branches of the caudal superficial epigastric vein are incised and ligated during dissection of tissues lateral to the prepuce.

C. Slight lateral retraction of the prepuce and incision of the subcutaneous tissue expose the linea alba and the external fascia of the rectus abdominis muscle. A stay suture is placed in the protractor preputii muscle to facilitate its identification during wound closure. The abdominal cavity is entered by tenting the abdominal wall cranially, after which the linea alba is sharply incised. Extension of the incision is performed by using a scalpel or scissors.

CLOSURE

The abdominal wall is closed with synthetic absorbable suture in a simple interrupted pattern. Subcutaneous tissue and the protractor preputii muscle are apposed with absorbable suture in a continuous or interrupted pattern. The skin is closed with nonabsorbable suture in a simple interrupted pattern.

COMMENTS

In the caudal portion of the abdomen, the linea alba becomes thin and when incised tends to retract, exposing muscle fibers of the rectus abdominis muscle. Proper closure technique includes engaging only the external rectus abdominis muscle fascia and not the muscle fibers when closing the caudal aspect of the incision.

The linea alba may be closed with a simple continuous pattern using synthetic nonabsorbable suture.

Plate 54

Approach to the Abdomen by Caudoventral Midline Celiotomy in the Male Dog *continued*

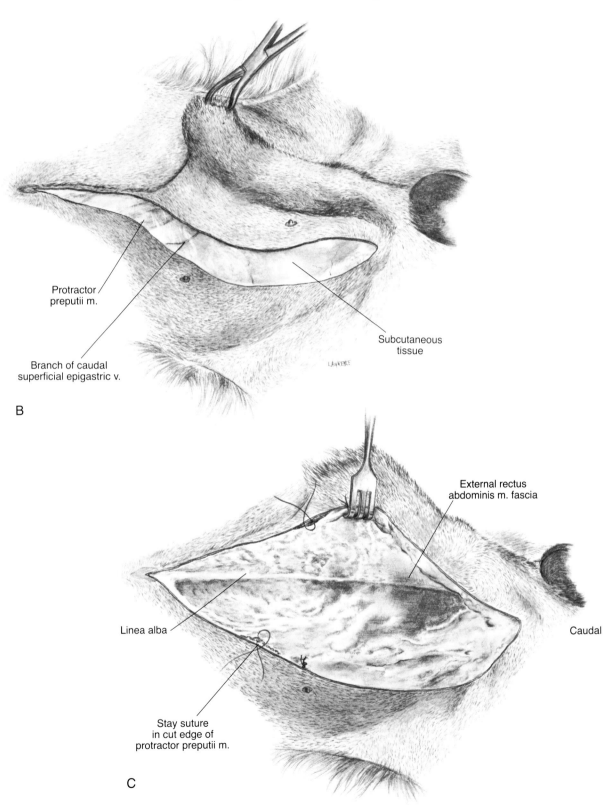

Protractor preputii m.

Subcutaneous tissue

Branch of caudal superficial epigastric v.

B

External rectus abdominis m. fascia

Linea alba

Caudal

Stay suture in cut edge of protractor preputii m.

C

Approach to the Abdomen by Paralumbar Celiotomy

INDICATIONS

Renal biopsy, adrenalectomy, ovariohysterectomy, and diseases involving the right or left craniolateral abdomen and retroperitoneal space.

DESCRIPTION OF THE PROCEDURE

A. The patient is positioned in lateral recumbency, with a rolled towel placed between the animal and the operating table. A skin incision is made from the ventral vertebral column to within 2 to 3 cm of the ventral midline. The incision is centered approximately halfway between the wing of the ilium and the last rib.

B. The incision is continued through the external abdominal oblique muscle to the caudoventral fibers of the internal abdominal oblique muscle.

Plate 55

Approach to the Abdomen by Paralumbar Celiotomy

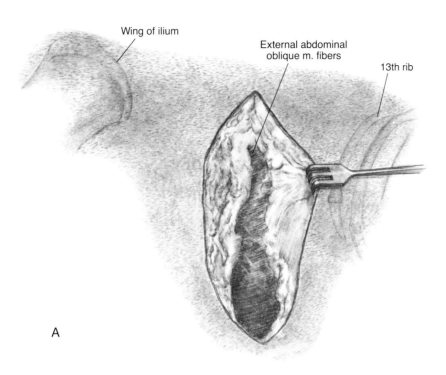

Wing of ilium

External abdominal
oblique m. fibers

13th rib

A

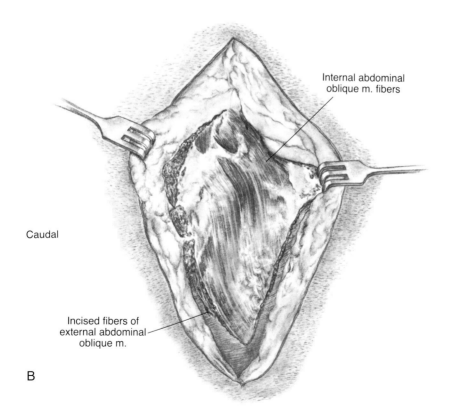

Internal abdominal
oblique m. fibers

Caudal

Incised fibers of
external abdominal
oblique m.

B

Approach to the Abdomen by Paralumbar Celiotomy *continued*

DESCRIPTION OF THE PROCEDURE *continued*

C. The internal abdominal oblique and the transversus abdominis muscle fibers are separated to expose the peritoneum and the transversalis fascia.

D. The peritoneal cavity is entered by tenting the peritoneum, after which a sharp incision is made with a scalpel. Digital exploration of the abdomen aids in locating the kidney, which is usually surrounded by abundant perirenal fat.

CLOSURE

Individual muscle layers of the incision are closed with synthetic absorbable suture in a continuous or interrupted pattern. Subcutaneous tissue is apposed with absorbable suture in a continuous or interrupted pattern. The skin is closed with nonabsorbable suture in a simple interrupted pattern.

COMMENTS

This approach has been used most commonly for renal biopsy.

Some surgeons believe that this is the approach of choice for adrenalectomy.

A more caudal location of the incision has been used extensively for ovariohysterectomy of the feline in the United Kingdom.

Plate 55

Approach to the Abdomen by Paralumbar
Celiotomy *continued*

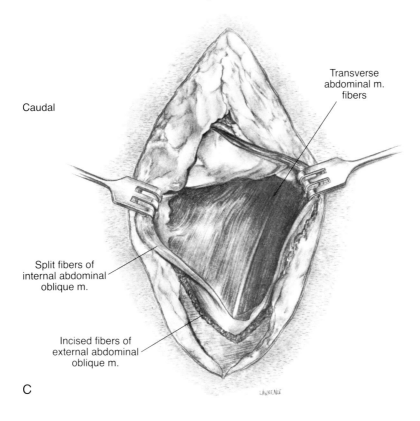

Caudal

Transverse
abdominal m.
fibers

Split fibers of
internal abdominal
oblique m.

Incised fibers of
external abdominal
oblique m.

C

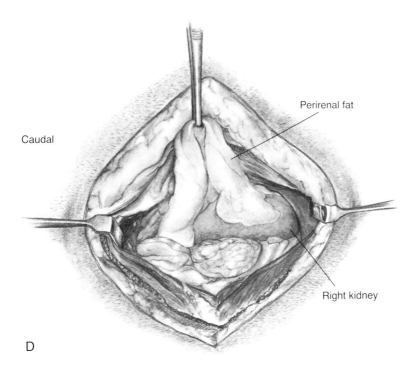

Caudal

Perirenal fat

Right kidney

D

Approach to the Esophageal Hiatus

INDICATIONS

Herniorraphy for gastroesophageal reflux and esophagitis secondary to hiatal hernia.

DESCRIPTION OF THE PROCEDURE

A. The patient is positioned in dorsal recumbency, and the abdomen is approached by cranioventral midline celiotomy (see p 166). Moistened laparotomy pads are placed to protect the abdominal wall, and self-retaining retractors are used to maintain visualization of the cranial abdominal viscera. The left lateral and medial lobes of the liver are retracted medially to expose the esophageal hiatus, which is located just dorsal to the central tendon of the diaphragm.

B. A stay suture is placed in the gastric fundus, and the stomach is retracted caudally. The phrenoesophageal membrane is incised around the periphery of the hiatus, with care being taken to avoid the dorsal and ventral vagus nerves.

C. Hiatal herniorraphy is performed by placing nonabsorbable suture in an interrupted mattress pattern through the right and left pars lumbalis of the diaphragmatic crura dorsal and ventral to the esophagus. The hiatus is closed to a diameter of 1.5 cm, permitting passage of an index finger through the hiatus. A permanent gastropexy is performed by attaching the gastric fundus to the left abdominal wall.

CLOSURE

The abdomen is closed as described in Approach to the Abdomen by Cranioventral Midline Celiotomy (see p 168).

COMMENTS

Incising the phrenoesophageal membrane creates a pneumothorax, requiring positive-pressure ventilation. Negative intrathoracic pressure should be reestablished prior to abdominal closure by thoracentesis using a needle or a soft rubber catheter and a three-way stopcock.

The need for an antireflux surgical procedure in addition to hiatal closure and gastropexy is controversial. The Nissen fundoplication technique, which consists of wrapping the gastroesophageal junction and the terminal 4 cm of esophagus with gastric fundus and suturing the fundus to itself, has been used successfully in the dog.

Based on a procedure of Ellison GW, Lewis DD, Phillips L, and Tarvin G: Esophageal hiatal hernia in small animals: literature review and a modified surgical technique. J Am Anim Hosp Assoc 23:391, 1987.

Plate 56

Approach to the Esophageal Hiatus

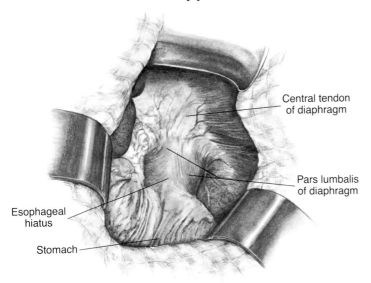

Central tendon
of diaphragm

Pars lumbalis
of diaphragm

Esophageal
hiatus

Stomach

A

Caudal

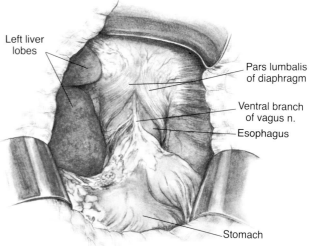

Left liver
lobes

Pars lumbalis
of diaphragm

Ventral branch
of vagus n.

Esophagus

Stomach

B

Caudal

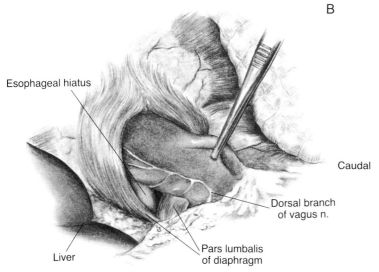

Esophageal hiatus

Caudal

Dorsal branch
of vagus n.

Pars lumbalis
of diaphragm

Liver

C

Approach to the Stomach

INDICATIONS

Gastrotomy for foreign body removal, partial gastrectomy for neoplasia or vascular compromise secondary to gastric volvulus, and gastropexy procedures performed at the pyloric antrum.

DESCRIPTION OF THE PROCEDURE

A. The patient is positioned in dorsal recumbency, and the abdomen is approached by cranioventral midline celiotomy (see p 166). Moistened laparotomy pads are placed to protect the abdominal wall, and self-retaining retractors are used to maintain visualization of the abdominal cavity. Adequate exposure is gained by caudal retraction of the greater curvature of the stomach.

B. Additional moistened laparotomy pads are placed to protect the abdominal viscera and to isolate the stomach. Traction stay sutures are placed to facilitate atraumatic tissue handling, and a gastrotomy is performed in a relatively avascular area midway between the greater and lesser curvatures of the stomach.

CLOSURE

Following foreign body removal or gastric wall resection, the gastric mucosa is closed with synthetic absorbable suture in a simple continuous pattern. The seromuscular layer is closed with synthetic absorbable suture in a continuous or interrupted Lembert pattern. The abdomen is lavaged copiously with warm saline and closed as described in Approach to the Abdomen by Cranioventral Midline Celiotomy (see p 168).

COMMENTS

Electrolyte and acid-base abnormalities are corrected prior to anesthesia and monitored postoperatively.

A complete exploration of the gastrointestinal tract is recommended to assure that all foreign bodies are identified.

A permanent gastropexy technique is indicated if surgery is performed for gastric volvulus.

Plate 57

Approach to the Stomach

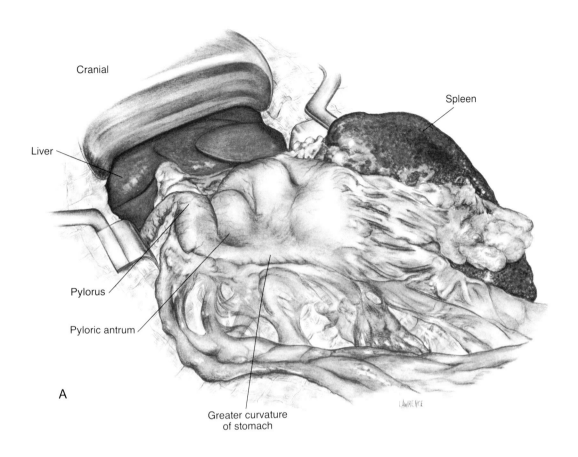

Cranial

Spleen

Liver

Pylorus

Pyloric antrum

A

Greater curvature
of stomach

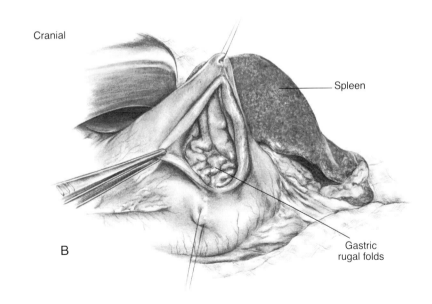

Cranial

Spleen

B

Gastric
rugal folds

Approach to the Pylorus

INDICATIONS

Enterotomy for foreign body, pyloroplasty techniques for delayed gastric emptying, and gastroduodenostomy for gastric ulcer or neoplasia.

DESCRIPTION OF THE PROCEDURE

A. The patient is positioned in dorsal recumbency and the abdomen is approached by cranioventral midline celiotomy (see p 166). Moistened laparotomy pads are placed to protect the abdominal wall, and self-retaining retractors are used to maintain visualization of the abdominal cavity. The pylorus is found in the right ventral abdominal quadrant in the normal dog and is relatively fixed in position by the hepatogastric and hepatoduodenal ligaments.

Plate 58

Approach to the Pylorus

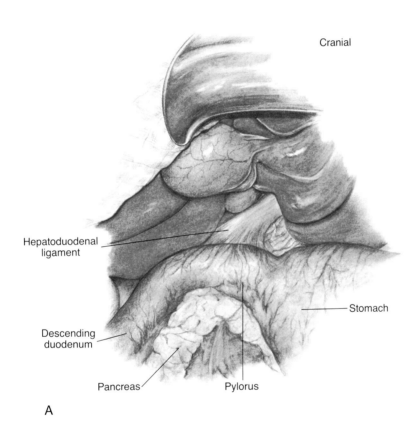

Cranial

Hepatoduodenal ligament

Stomach

Descending duodenum

Pancreas

Pylorus

A

Approach to the Pylorus *continued*

DESCRIPTION OF THE PROCEDURE *continued*

B. Gastroduodenostomy is initiated by isolation and ligation of the right gastric artery, which courses in the lesser omentum on the cranial aspect of the pylorus. On the greater curvature, blunt dissection is used to isolate branches of the right gastro-epiploic artery close to the serosal surface of the stomach. The extent of resection is determined by the operative goals and the area of diseased tissue. Care is taken to preserve the bile duct distally.

C. Atraumatic intestinal clamps are positioned at the site of resection, and partial gastrectomy is performed. The point of resection is higher on the lesser curvature than on the greater curvature to avoid formation of a blind sac at the anastomotic site. The gastric stump is closed with synthetic absorbable suture, leaving a stoma that is the same size as the duodenal stoma.

CLOSURE

Gastroduodenal anastomosis is completed by using synthetic absorbable suture in a simple interrupted pattern between the gastric and duodenal stomas. The abdomen is lavaged copiously with warm saline and closed as described in Approach to the Abdomen by Cranioventral Midline Celiotomy (see p 168).

COMMENTS

The approach and surgical procedure described (Billroth I) are most appropriate for animals with benign obstructive disease (hypertrophic pyloric gastropathy) or gastric ulceration. Gastric ulcers may be caused by oral medications, mast cell neoplasia, and rarely neoplasia of the pancreas.

Y-U pyloroplasty is an effective surgical procedure for some patients with hypertrophic pyloric gastropathy.

Plate 58

Approach to the Pylorus *continued*

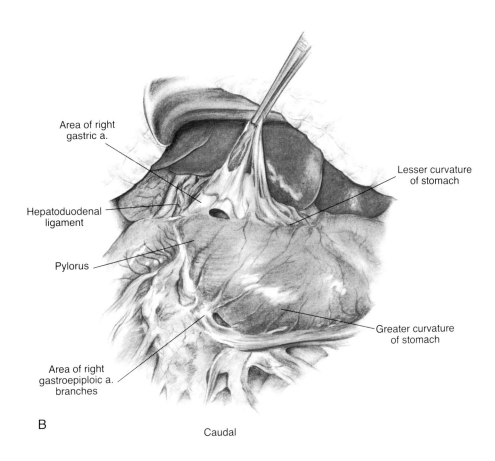

Area of right
gastric a.

Lesser curvature
of stomach

Hepatoduodenal
ligament

Pylorus

Greater curvature
of stomach

Area of right
gastroepiploic a.
branches

B

Caudal

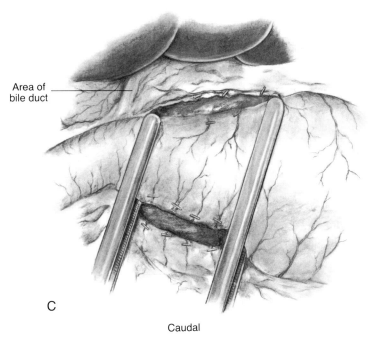

Area of
bile duct

C

Caudal

Approach to the Pancreas

INDICATIONS

Pancreatic biopsy, pancreatic lavage and drainage, and partial or total pancreatectomy for neoplasia.

DESCRIPTION OF THE PROCEDURE

A. The patient is positioned in dorsal recumbency, and the abdomen is approached by cranioventral midline celiotomy (see p 166). Moistened laparotomy pads are placed to protect the abdominal wall, and self-retaining retractors are used to maintain visualization of the cranial abdominal viscera. The pancreas lies in close association with the duodenum, the pylorus, and the stomach. The left lobe of the pancreas runs dorsally and obliquely to the left in the greater omentum, ending in the left sublumbar region close to the aorta and the left kidney.

B. The right lobe of the pancreas is exposed by ventromedial retraction of the duodenum. Blood supply to the cranial half of the right lobe is from the cranial pancreaticoduodenal artery. This artery courses within the pancreatic parenchyma before leaving the gland to lie on the mesenteric border of the duodenum, where it anastomoses with the caudal pancreaticoduodenal artery. Branches of these arteries supply the duodenum as well as the pancreas. Preservation of these vessels during pancreatic surgery minimizes the risk of vascular compromise to the duodenum caused by surgery.

Plate 59

Approach to the Pancreas

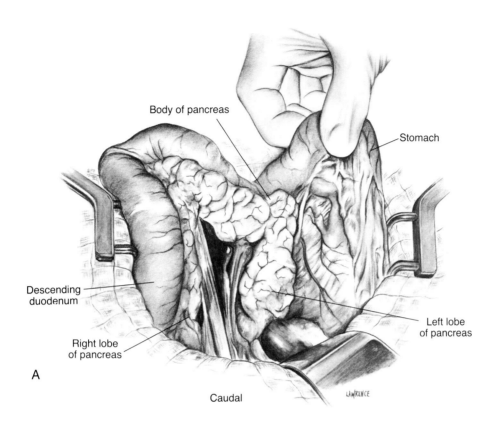

Body of pancreas

Stomach

Descending
duodenum

Left lobe
of pancreas

Right lobe
of pancreas

A

Caudal

LAWRENCE

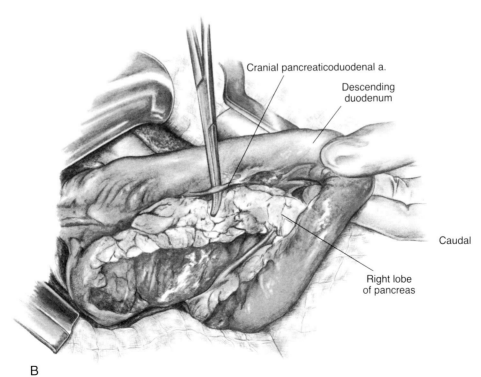

Cranial pancreaticoduodenal a.

Descending
duodenum

Caudal

Right lobe
of pancreas

B

Approach to the Pancreas *continued*

DESCRIPTION OF THE PROCEDURE *continued*

C. Pancreatic biopsy is performed at the caudal aspect of the gland to avoid disruption of major ducts. The mesoduodenum is fenestrated, and absorbable suture is used to isolate and ligate the distal pancreas before excision.

CLOSURE

The fenestrated mesoduodenum is closed with a continuous pattern of absorbable suture. The abdomen is closed as described in Approach to the Abdomen by Cranioventral Midline Celiotomy (see p 168).

COMMENTS

The left pancreatic lobe is less mobile than the right, making surgical exposure more difficult. Retraction of the stomach cranially and use of the colon and mesocolon to retract the small intestine caudally aids exposure of the left lobe. The greater omentum may be fenestrated to further expose the ventral surface of the left lobe.

Damage to the cranial pancreaticoduodenal artery may result in duodenal ischemia, requiring intestinal resection and anastomosis.

Total pancreatectomy with or without duodenectomy is a formidable surgical procedure that is rarely indicated in the dog.

Gentle tissue handling may decrease the incidence of postoperative pancreatitis and ileus.

Plate 59

Approach to the Pancreas *continued*

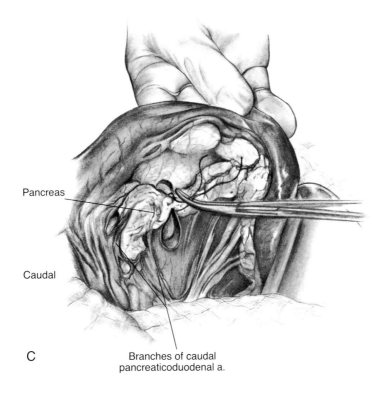

Pancreas

Caudal

C   Branches of caudal
     pancreaticoduodenal a.

Approach to the Small Intestine

INDICATIONS

Exploration of the gastrointestinal tract, enterotomy for biopsy or foreign body removal, and intestinal resection and anastomosis.

DESCRIPTION OF THE PROCEDURE

A. The patient is positioned in dorsal recumbency, and the abdomen is approached by cranioventral midline celiotomy (see p 166). The incision is extended caudally as necessary to allow complete examination of the gastrointestinal tract. Moistened laparotomy pads are placed to protect the abdominal wall, and self-retaining retractors are used to maintain visualization of the abdominal cavity. The duodenum begins at the pylorus in the right cranial abdominal quadrant and extends caudally. The duodenum is relatively fixed cranially by the hepatoduodenal ligament, which contains the bile duct extending from the liver to the duodenum.

Plate 60

Approach to the Small Intestine

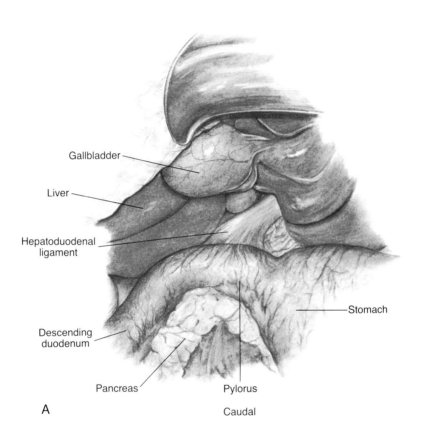

Gallbladder

Liver

Hepatoduodenal ligament

Descending duodenum

Pancreas

Pylorus

Stomach

A

Caudal

Approach to the Small Intestine *continued*

DESCRIPTION OF THE PROCEDURE *continued*

B. The descending duodenum and the right limb of the pancreas may be partially exteriorized and examined. Ventromedial retraction of the duodenum and the mesoduodenum results in displacement of the viscera to the left, allowing examination of the right kidney, the ureter, and the ovary, if desired.

C. The duodenum makes a U-shaped turn caudally and ascends ventrocaudally to the stomach, where the jejunum begins. Exposure and exteriorization of the duodenum at its caudal flexure are more difficult because of the short duodenocolic ligament. Exposure is facilitated by incision of the ligament.

Plate 60

Approach to the Small Intestine *continued*

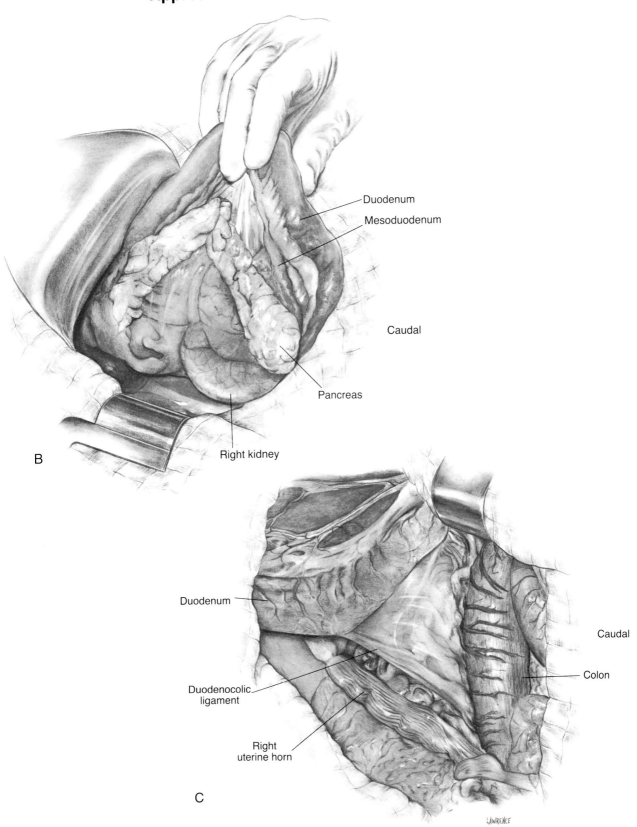

B

Duodenum
Mesoduodenum
Caudal
Pancreas
Right kidney

C

Duodenum
Caudal
Colon
Duodenocolic ligament
Right uterine horn

LAWRENCE

Approach to the Small Intestine *continued*

DESCRIPTION OF THE PROCEDURE *continued*

D. Most of the small intestine is composed of jejunum and ileum. The jejunum and ileum are the most mobile parts of the gastrointestinal tract and are easily exteriorized. Blood supply to the jejunum is via 12 to 15 jejunal arteries and veins that traverse the mesojejunum. The ileum is the terminal part of the small intestine and may be recognized by the presence of the antimesenteric ileal branch of the ileocolic artery and the presence of the ileocecal fold between the ileum and cecum.

E. The ileocolic junction marks the boundary between the small intestine and the large intestine. Mesenteric lymph nodes are often prominent and well visualized in this area.

CLOSURE

The abdomen is closed as described in Approach to the Abdomen by Cranioventral Midline Celiotomy (see p 168).

COMMENTS

The entire gastrointestinal tract should be thoroughly explored prior to definitive surgery.

The intestinal serosa is normally a glistening pink color. Clinical criteria for intestinal viability are color, peristalsis, and arterial pulsations.

The ileocolic junction is a common location of intussusception.

Lymph node biopsy is easily performed on mesenteric lymph nodes; care is taken to not disturb vasculature supplying intestine.

Plate 60

Approach to the Small Intestine *continued*

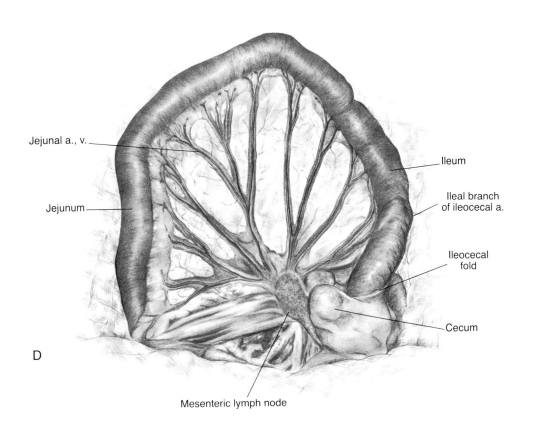

Jejunal a., v.

Jejunum

Ileum

Ileal branch
of ileocecal a.

Ileocecal
fold

Cecum

Mesenteric lymph node

D

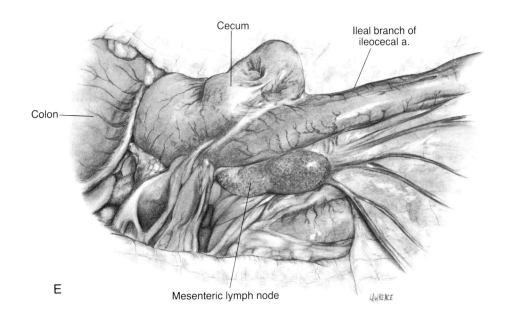

Cecum

Ileal branch of
ileocecal a.

Colon

Mesenteric lymph node

E

Approach to the Colon

INDICATIONS

Biopsy and resection and anastomosis for neoplastic disease and idiopathic megacolon.

DESCRIPTION OF THE PROCEDURE

A. The patient is positioned in dorsal recumbency, and the abdomen is approached by caudoventral midline celiotomy, with specific techniques depending on the sex of the patient (see p 172 or p 174). Moistened laparotomy pads are placed to protect the abdominal wall, and self-retaining retractors are used to maintain visualization of the abdominal cavity. The colon begins at the ileocolic sphincter and, as compared with the small intestine, is characterized by a larger diameter and a relatively segmental blood supply. Caudally, the colon enters the pelvic inlet, where it continues as the rectum to terminate at the anus. Blood supply to the colon cranially is via ileocolic and middle colic branches of the cranial mesenteric artery and caudally from the left colic artery, a branch of the caudal mesenteric artery. In preparation for colectomy, the colic and caudal mesenteric vessels supplying the segment of colon to be excised are ligated and transected. Caudally, the colon is excised 2 to 3 cm cranial to the pecten ossis pubis, facilitating anastomosis without pelvic osteotomy.

B. The ileocolic junction is resected in cases of idiopathic megacolon and in many cases of intussusception necessitating an ileocolic anastomosis. Luminal size disparity between the ileum and the colon is corrected by partial closure of the colon with synthetic absorbable suture in an inverting pattern. Anastomosis is completed by placement of simple interrupted appositional sutures between the ileum and the colon.

CLOSURE

The mesenteric defect is closed with absorbable suture in a continuous pattern. The abdomen is closed as described in the caudoventral Approach to the Abdomen by Caudoventral Midline Celiotomy (see p 172 or p 176).

COMMENTS

Neoplastic disease involving the caudal colon and the rectum may require resection of the pubis to provide adequate surgical exposure for resection and anastomosis (see p 202). Resection and anastomosis of the caudal and intrapelvic colon are enhanced by the use of surgical stapling equipment.

Subtotal colectomy is recommended in cats for treatment of idiopathic megacolon that is unresponsive to medical therapy. Other methods of correcting intestinal luminal disparity include incising the smaller diameter bowel at an angle and/or incising the antimesenteric border longitudinally.

Perioperative prophylactic antibiotics effective against both aerobic and anaerobic bacteria are indicated for patients undergoing colonic surgery.

Plate 61

Approach to the Colon

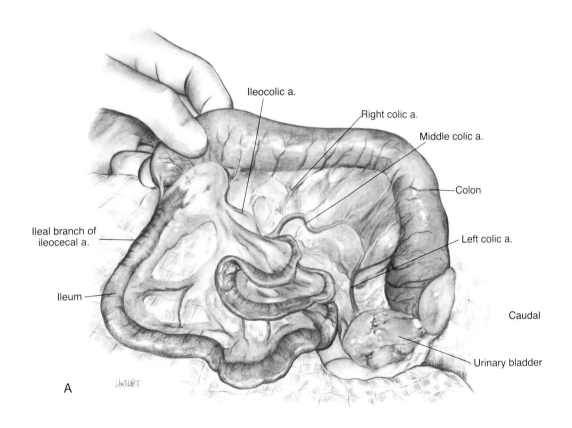

Ileocolic a.

Right colic a.

Middle colic a.

Colon

Left colic a.

Ileal branch of
ileocecal a.

Ileum

Caudal

Urinary bladder

A

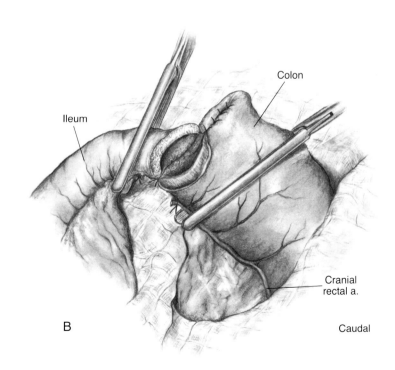

Ileum

Colon

Cranial
rectal a.

B

Caudal

Approach to the Pelvic Canal

INDICATIONS

Surgical exposure of the prostate, the pelvic urethra, and the caudal colon and rectum.

DESCRIPTION OF THE PROCEDURE

A. The patient is positioned in dorsal recumbency, and the abdomen is approached by caudoventral midline celiotomy, with specific techniques depending on the sex of the patient (see p 172 or p 174). The skin incision is extended caudally over the pelvic midline to the caudal aspect of the pubis. Subcutaneous tissues are incised to expose the ventral pelvic musculature.

B. The approach is continued by sharp dissection of the gracilis and adductor muscles on the midline. The adductor muscles are elevated subperiosteally from medial to lateral, exposing the obturator nerve and approximately half of the obturator foramen. Holes are drilled on each aspect of the proposed osteotomy sites (dotted lines), and osteotomy is performed by using a Gigli-saw wire, an osteotome, or an oscillating saw.

C. The internal obturator muscle is subperiosteally elevated from the left pubis and the ischium, allowing retraction of the central pubic segment to the right. Fatty tissue is bluntly dissected to expose the intrapelvic viscera.

CLOSURE

The pubic segment is cerclaged using stainless steel wire. The adductor and gracilis muscles are reapposed with absorbable suture in a continuous or interrupted pattern. The abdomen is closed as described in Approach to the Abdomen by Caudoventral Midline Celiotomy (see p 172 or p 176).

COMMENTS

Most animals are totally ambulatory within 24 hours. Postoperative exercise is limited to leash walks for 8 weeks.

Based on a procedure of Allen SW, and Crowell WA: Ventral approach to the pelvic canal in the female dog. Vet Surg 20:118, 1991.

Plate 62

Approach to the Pelvic Canal

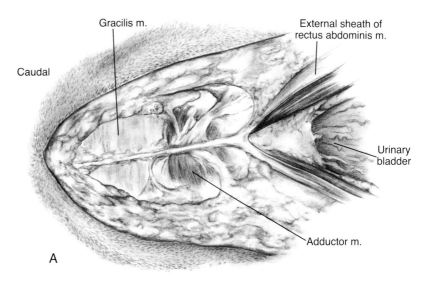

A

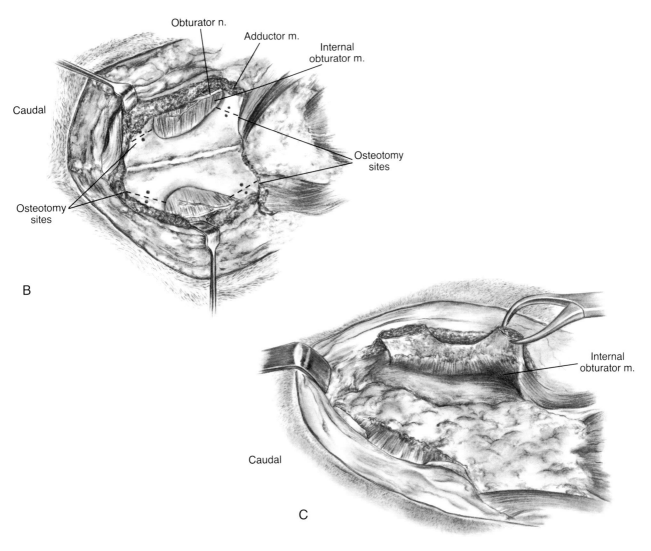

B

C

Approach to the Pelvic Canal and the Rectum (Dorsal)

INDICATIONS

Surgical treatment of rectal tear, perianal fistula, rectal stricture or diverticula, rectal neoplasia, neoplasia of the dorsal pelvic canal, and bilateral perineal herniorrhaphy.

DESCRIPTION OF THE PROCEDURE

A. The patient is positioned in ventral recumbency, with the pelvis elevated and the tail positioned craniodorsally and taped in place. The area below the proximal hindlimb is padded to prevent pressure on the femoral nerve. A purse-string suture is placed in the anus to prevent fecal contamination of the operative field. A U-shaped skin incision is made between the tail base and the anus connecting the perineal areas.

B. Subcutaneous tissue and fat are incised to expose the rectococcygeus, the levator ani, and the coccygeus muscles. The external anal sphincter and the rectum also should be identified. The rectococcygeus muscle is bluntly undermined and incised near its insertion on the caudal vertebrae.

Plate 63

Approach to the Pelvic Canal and the Rectum (Dorsal)

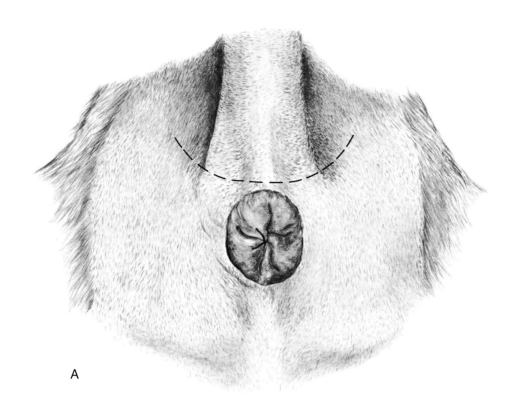

A

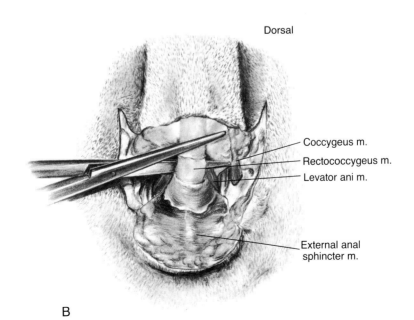

Dorsal

Coccygeus m.

Rectococcygeus m.

Levator ani m.

External anal
sphincter m.

B

Approach to the Pelvic Canal and the Rectum
(Dorsal) *continued*

DESCRIPTION OF THE PROCEDURE *continued*

C. A stay suture is used to aid ventrolateral retraction of the rectococcygeus muscle. Increased exposure of the rectum may be gained by bluntly separating the caudal aspect of the levator ani muscles from the external anal sphincter and/or by myotomy of the levator ani muscles.

D. The levator ani muscles are incised bilaterally perpendicular to their fibers; care is taken to preserve the caudal rectal nerve and the peritoneal reflection.

CLOSURE

The rectococcygeus muscle is reattached with synthetic absorbable suture in an interrupted cruciate or other mattress pattern. Incised borders of the levator ani muscles are apposed with synthetic absorbable suture in an interrupted pattern. A Penrose or closed-suction drainage system may be placed in the perirectal area following extensive lavage with isotonic fluid. The subcutaneous tissues are apposed with absorbable suture in a continuous or interrupted pattern, and the skin is closed with nonabsorbable suture in an interrupted pattern.

COMMENTS

The urethra should be identified by catheterization if extensive dissection is expected.

Transection of the levator ani muscles may not be necessary for procedures requiring limited exposure.

Length of rectal resection should be limited to 4 cm to preserve normal fecal continence. Rectal resection cranial to or involving a large portion of the peritoneal reflection may result in fecal incontinence.

Based on a procedure of McKeown DB, Cockshutt JR, Partlow GD, and de Kleer VS: Dorsal approach to the caudal pelvic canal and rectum: effect on normal dogs. Vet Surg 13:181, 1984.

Plate 63

Approach to the Pelvic Canal and the Rectum
(Dorsal) *continued*

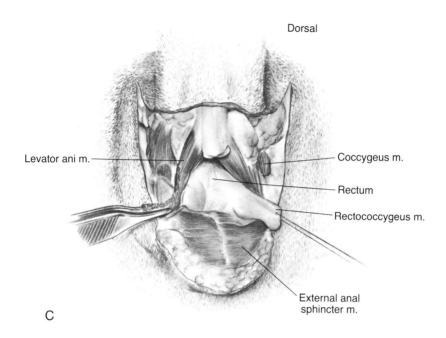

Dorsal

Levator ani m.

Coccygeus m.

Rectum

Rectococcygeus m.

External anal
sphincter m.

C

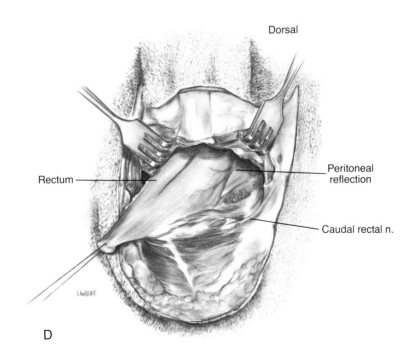

Dorsal

Rectum

Peritoneal
reflection

Caudal rectal n.

LAWRENCE

D

Approach to the Spleen

INDICATIONS

Splenectomy for neoplasia and partial splenectomy for trauma or biopsy.

DESCRIPTION OF THE PROCEDURE

A. The patient is positioned in dorsal recumbency, and the abdomen is approached by cranioventral midline celiotomy (see p 166). The spleen, which is located in the left cranial abdominal quadrant, is exteriorized and packed off with moistened laparotomy pads. The splenic and left gastroepiploic arteries are identified as they course through the greater omentum and the gastrosplenic ligament. Splenectomy is performed by double ligation and severance of numerous splenic hilar vessels with absorbable suture material.

B. Splenectomy may be facilitated by use of surgical stapling equipment (Ligating-Dividing Stapler [LDS], U.S. Surgical Corporation, Norwalk, CT) or vascular clips instead of ligatures.

Plate 64
Approach to the Spleen

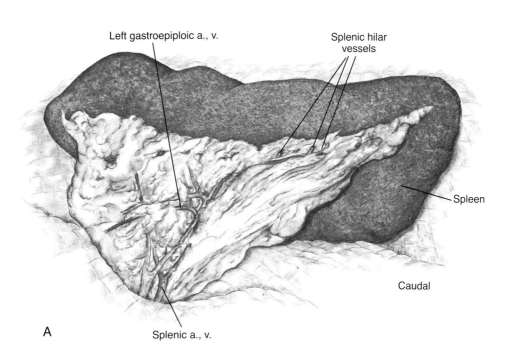

Left gastroepiploic a., v.

Splenic hilar vessels

Spleen

Caudal

A

Splenic a., v.

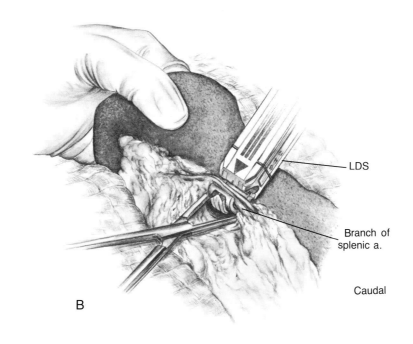

LDS

Branch of splenic a.

Caudal

B

Approach to the Spleen *continued*

DESCRIPTION OF THE PROCEDURE *continued*

C. Partial splenectomy is performed by ligating or stapling hilar vessels supplying the portion of the spleen to be excised. The splenic parenchyma is digitally "milked" toward the splenic segment to be excised prior to placement of the thoracoabdominal stapling instrument (TA-55, U.S. Surgical Corporation, Norwalk, CT) at the excision site. After proper instrument placement, the staples are fired and the spleen is excised by scalpel, using the instrument as a cutting guide. Alternatively, atraumatic intestinal forceps are placed at the excision site, and the splenic capsule is oversewn with a continuous pattern of absorbable suture (inset).

CLOSURE

The abdomen is closed as described in Approach to the Abdomen by Cranioventral Midline Celiotomy (see p 168).

COMMENTS

The left gastroepiploic artery provides vascular supply to the greater curvature of the stomach and should be preserved. Ligation of the short gastric arteries may be performed if necessary.

When total splenectomy is performed with ligatures, some surgeons recommend inversion of the greater omentum with absorbable suture and a continuous suture pattern to reduce the incidence of adhesion of abdominal viscera to exposed suture.

Prior to abdominal closure, adequate hemostasis is assured by inspecting the greater omentum after splenectomy or the remaining spleen after partial splenectomy.

The authors believe that the use of epinephrine to decrease splenic size by inducing splenic contraction is contraindicated.

Plate 64

Approach to the Spleen *continued*

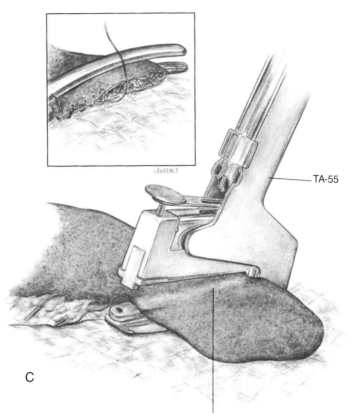

TA-55

C

Line of demarcation between
perfused and ischemic spleen

Approach to the Hepatic Veins

INDICATIONS

Attenuation of the left hepatic vein as treatment for intrahepatic portosystemic shunt involving the left liver lobes and intravascular attenuation of intrahepatic portosystemic shunts.

DESCRIPTION OF THE PROCEDURE

A. The patient is positioned in dorsal recumbency, and the abdomen is approached by cranioventral midline celiotomy (see p 166). Moistened laparotomy pads are placed to protect the abdominal wall, and self-retaining retractors are used to maintain visualization of cranial abdominal viscera.

B. The left lateral and medial liver lobes and the stomach are retracted caudally and protected with moistened laparotomy pads. The left triangular ligament attaching the left lobe of the liver to the diaphragm is incised to facilitate exposure of the hepatic veins.

C. The left hepatic vein, the most cranially located hepatic vein, enters the left ventral aspect of the caudal vena cava. Using blunt dissection, the left hepatic vein is carefully isolated (inset), and moistened silk suture is positioned to be used in partial or complete attentuation of the vessel.

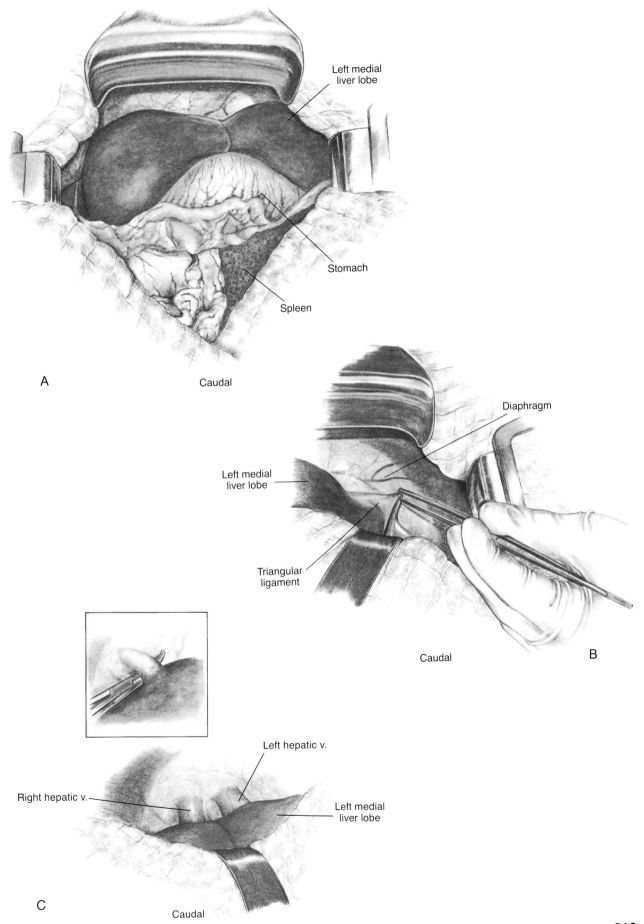

A

Left medial liver lobe

Stomach

Spleen

Caudal

B

Diaphragm

Left medial liver lobe

Triangular ligament

Caudal

C

Left hepatic v.

Right hepatic v.

Left medial liver lobe

Caudal

213

Approach to the Hepatic Veins *continued*

DESCRIPTION OF THE PROCEDURE *continued*

D. Intravascular repair of portosystemic shunts is performed via venotomy in the intrathoracic caudal vena cava. A cranioventral midline celiotomy incision is extended cranially through the last 3 to 4 sternebrae. The diaphragm is incised to the level of the caudal vena cava, and stay sutures are placed to aid exposure of the caudal vena cava. Prior to caval venotomy, the portal vein, the prehepatic caudal vena cava, the posthepatic vena cava, the celiac artery, and the cranial mesenteric artery are temporarily occluded with tourniquets or vascular clamps. An atraumatic vascular occlusion clamp is applied tangentially, and an incision is made in the vena cava.

E. Stay sutures are placed to aid intravascular exposure. The normal hepatic veins have smooth margins and a "tunneled" appearance.

CLOSURE

A continuous suture pattern using polypropylene is placed to close the venotomy incision. The sternebrae are apposed using nonabsorbable suture in a circumferential cruciate pattern. The abdomen is closed as described in Approach to the Abdomen by Cranioventral Midline Celiotomy (see p 168).

COMMENTS

Congenital intrahepatic portosystemic shunts are most often attributable to patent ductus venosus located in the left liver lobes. This vessel usually enters the left hepatic vein but may enter the caudal vena cava directly or be located in the right liver division. Portography performed by cannulation of the splenic or jejunal veins is recommended to verify shunt location and to measure portal pressure during shunt ligation.

Portal system pressure is measured during shunt attentuation to avoid the potential fatal postoperative complication of portal hypertension. Postligation portal pressure should not exceed 10 cm H_2O above preligation baseline values and should not exceed 20 cm H_2O in any case.

The urinary system is palpated for the presence of uroliths in animals with portosystemic shunts.

Based on procedures of Martin RA, and Freeman LE: Identification and surgical management of portosystemic shunts in the dog and cat. Vet Med Surg (Small Animal) 2:302, 1987; and Breznock EM, Berger B, Pendray D, et al: Surgical manipulation of intrahepatic portacaval shunts in dogs. J Am Vet Med Assoc 182:798, 1983.

Plate 65

Approach to the Hepatic Veins *continued*

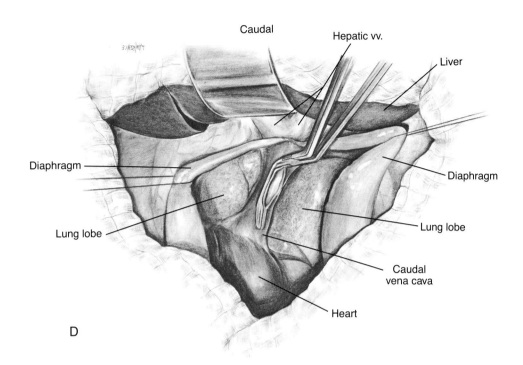

Caudal

Hepatic vv.

Liver

Diaphragm

Diaphragm

Lung lobe

Lung lobe

Caudal
vena cava

Heart

D

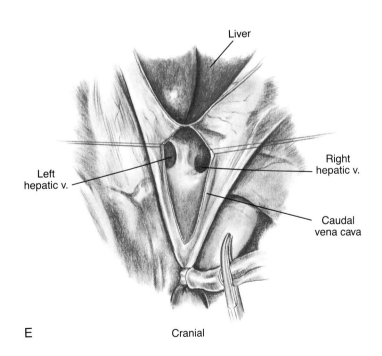

Liver

Left
hepatic v.

Right
hepatic v.

Caudal
vena cava

E

Cranial

Approach to the Epiploic Foramen

INDICATIONS

Exploratory surgery for portosystemic shunts and vascular occlusion to decrease hemorrhage from the liver.

DESCRIPTION OF THE PROCEDURE

A. The patient is positioned in dorsal recumbency, and the abdomen is approached by cranioventral midline celiotomy (see p 166). Moistened laparotomy pads are placed to protect the abdominal wall, and self-retaining retractors are used to maintain visualization of the abdominal cavity. Ventromedial retraction of the duodenum and mesoduodenum is used to expose the right craniodorsal abdomen.

B. The epiploic foramen is a 2- 3-cm opening into the lesser peritoneum craniomedial to the right kidney and medial to the caudate process of the liver. It is bounded by the caudal vena cava dorsally and the portal vein ventrally. A finger may be placed from lateral to medial through the foramen and curled ventrally to compress the blood supply to the liver from the hepatic artery and the portal vein.

Plate 66

Approach to the Epiploic Foramen

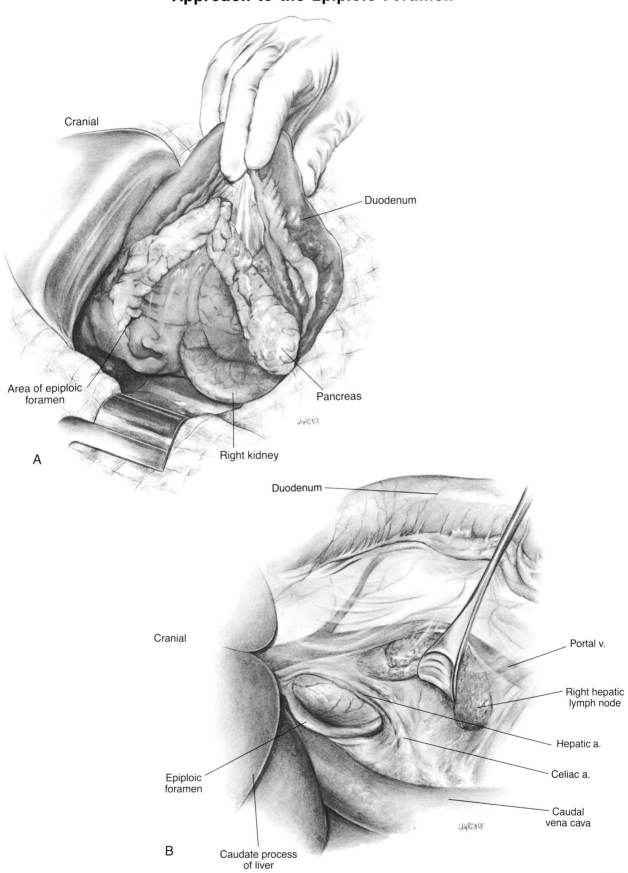

Cranial

Duodenum

Area of epiploic
foramen

Pancreas

Right kidney

A

Duodenum

Cranial

Portal v.

Right hepatic
lymph node

Hepatic a.

Celiac a.

Epiploic
foramen

Caudal
vena cava

B   Caudate process
of liver

217

Approach to the Epiploic Foramen *continued*

DESCRIPTION OF THE PROCEDURE *continued*

C. From a ventral approach, the omentum is fenestrated along its ventral aspect while the stomach is retracted cranially and the duodenum ventrally and to the right. The left gastric and splenic veins are identified medial to the junction of the splenic and portal veins. Most single extrahepatic portosystemic shunts arise from the splenic vein or the left gastric vein and extend to the caudal vena cava through the epiploic foramen.

CLOSURE

The abdomen is closed as described in Approach to the Abdomen by Cranioventral Midline Celiotomy (see p 168).

COMMENTS

Temporary occlusion of hepatic blood supply is helpful in controlling hemorrhage from massive liver injury. Vascular occlusion should be limited to 10 to 15 minutes, although this time period may be extended if occlusion is intermittent. Parenteral antibiotics are indicated in such cases owing to the normal microbial flora of the canine portohepatic circulation.

Knowledge of local anatomy may allow portosystemic shunt identification and attenuation without portography. Splenic or jejunal vein cannulation is performed to measure portal pressure during shunt ligation and is used for portography if necessary. Digital or ligature occlusion of the shunt will result in a rapid rise in portal pressure, helping confirm identification of the shunt. Postligation portal pressure should not exceed 10 cm H_2O above preligation baseline values and should not exceed 20 cm H_2O in any case.

The urinary system is palpated for the presence of uroliths in animals with portosystemic shunts.

Plate 66

Approach to the Epiploic Foramen *continued*

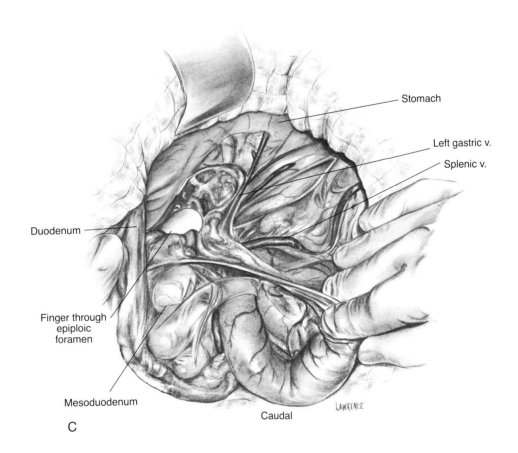

Stomach

Left gastric v.

Splenic v.

Duodenum

Finger through
epiploic
foramen

Mesoduodenum

Caudal

LAWRENCE

C

Approach to the Extrahepatic Biliary System

INDICATIONS

Cholecystectomy, cholecystoenterostomy, and exploration of the extrahepatic biliary system.

DESCRIPTION OF THE PROCEDURE

A. The patient is positioned in dorsal recumbency, and the abdomen is approached by cranioventral midline celiotomy (see p 166). Moistened laparotomy pads are placed to protect the abdominal wall, and self-retaining retractors are used to maintain visualization of the abdominal cavity. The pylorus and duodenum are relatively fixed in position by the hepatoduodenal ligament and the mesoduodenum, respectively.

B. Careful retraction of the duodenum and the stomach caudally and the liver cranially exposes the hepatoduodenal ligament, through which the bile duct courses from the liver to the duodenum. Numerous branches of the portal vein supply the liver lobes and may be encountered at the porta hepatis.

Plate 67

Approach to the Extrahepatic Biliary System

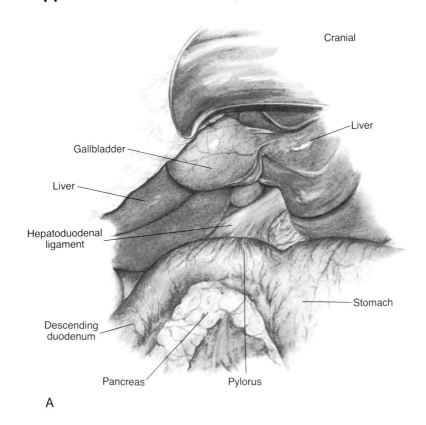

Cranial

Liver

Gallbladder

Liver

Hepatoduodenal
ligament

Descending
duodenum

Pancreas

Pylorus

Stomach

A

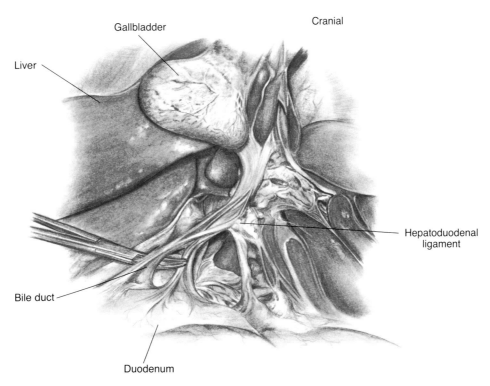

Gallbladder

Cranial

Liver

Hepatoduodenal
ligament

Bile duct

Duodenum

B

Approach to the Extrahepatic Biliary System *continued*

DESCRIPTION OF THE PROCEDURE *continued*

C. The bile duct receives bile-circulating tributaries from a variable number of hepatic ducts and the cystic duct from the gallbladder. The gallbladder lies in a fossa between the quadrate lobe medially and the right medial lobe laterally. The fundus of the gallbladder may be mobilized by sharp and blunt dissection of its fibrous attachments to the fossa of the right medial lobe. Hemostasis may be achieved using electrocautery or direct pressure with gauze sponges.

D. The terminal portion of the bile duct enters the dorsal or mesenteric wall of the duodenum and courses intramurally a short distance (1.5 to 2.0 cm) before opening on the major duodenal papilla. The papilla is located 3 to 6 cm from the pylorus and is exposed by enterotomy on the antimesenteric aspect of the duodenum. Stay sutures facilitate exposure of the papilla, which may be catheterized to confirm patency and integrity of the bile duct.

CLOSURE

If enterotomy is performed, it is closed with synthetic absorbable suture in a simple interrupted pattern. The abdomen is closed as described in Approach to the Abdomen by Cranioventral Midline Celiotomy (see p 168).

COMMENTS

Exploration of the extrahepatic biliary system is performed to identify neoplastic or inflammatory disease that may cause biliary obstruction. Gentle manual expression of the gallbladder may confirm patency of the cystic and common bile ducts.

When cholecystectomy is performed, the gallbladder is bluntly dissected from its fossa, and the cystic duct is ligated prior to its junction with the hepatic ducts.

Catheterization of the major duodenal papilla may be used to collect biliary fluid for bacterial culture. Suture repair of tears in the bile duct may be performed over the catheter.

Plate 67

Approach to the Extrahepatic Biliary System *continued*

Cranial

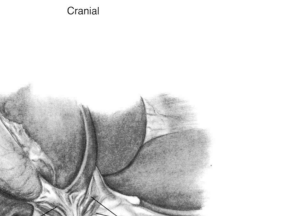

Gallbladder

Hepatic
ducts

Cystic
duct

C

Major duodenal
papilla

Duodenal lumen

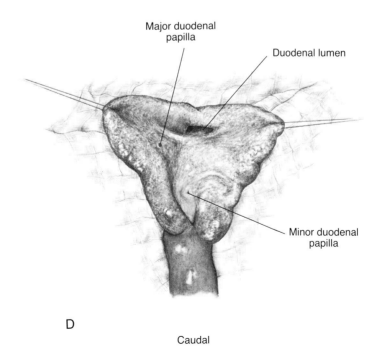

Minor duodenal
papilla

D

Caudal

Approach to the Adrenal Glands

INDICATIONS

Incisional or excisional biopsy of the adrenal glands for hyperplasia or neoplasia.

DESCRIPTION OF THE PROCEDURE

A. The patient is positioned in dorsal recumbency, and the abdomen is approached by cranioventral midline celiotomy (see p 166). Moistened laparotomy pads are placed to protect the abdominal wall, and self-retaining retractors are used to maintain visualization of the abdominal cavity. Ventromedial retraction of the descending colon and the mesocolon is used to pack abdominal viscera to the right, exposing the left kidney and the retroperitoneal space.

Plate 68

Approach to the Adrenal Glands

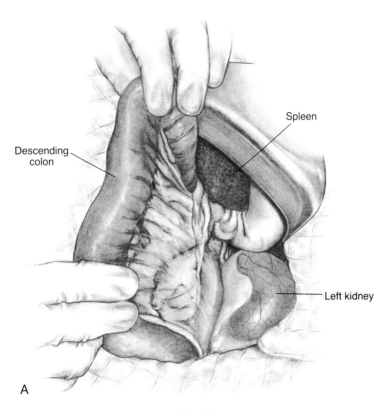

Spleen

Descending
colon

Left kidney

A

Caudal

Approach to the Adrenal Glands *continued*

DESCRIPTION OF THE PROCEDURE *continued*

B. The spleen and the stomach are packed off cranially with moistened laparotomy pads, further exposing the left retroperitoneal space cranial to the left kidney. The phrenicoabdominal vein is visualized coursing over the ventral surface of the left adrenal gland, which is located craniomedial to the left kidney. The oval cranial portion of the gland is more easily visualized than the caudal aspect, which may be obscured by varying amounts of fatty tissue.

C. A combination of blunt and sharp dissection of surrounding fatty tissue is used to fully expose the adrenal gland. Care is taken in caudal dissection to avoid the renal artery and vein. The phrenicoabdominal artery courses over the dorsomedial aspect of the gland. Isolation and ligation of the phrenicoabdominal artery and vein with synthetic absorbable suture are necessary if adrenalectomy is performed.

Plate 68

Approach to the Adrenal Glands *continued*

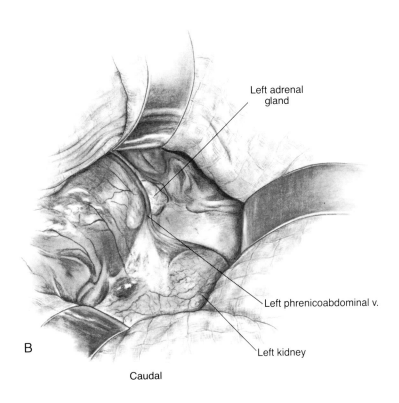

Left adrenal
gland

Left phrenicoabdominal v.

Left kidney

B

Caudal

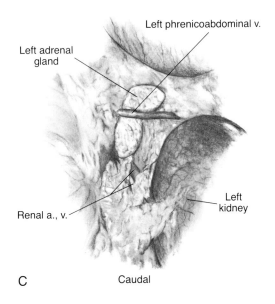

Left phrenicoabdominal v.

Left adrenal
gland

Left
kidney

Renal a., v.

C

Caudal

Approach to the Adrenal Glands *continued*

DESCRIPTION OF THE PROCEDURE *continued*

D. To expose the right adrenal gland, ventromedial retraction of the duodenum and the mesoduodenum is used to pack abdominal viscera to the left, exposing the right kidney and the retroperitoneal space.

Plate 68

Approach to the Adrenal Glands *continued*

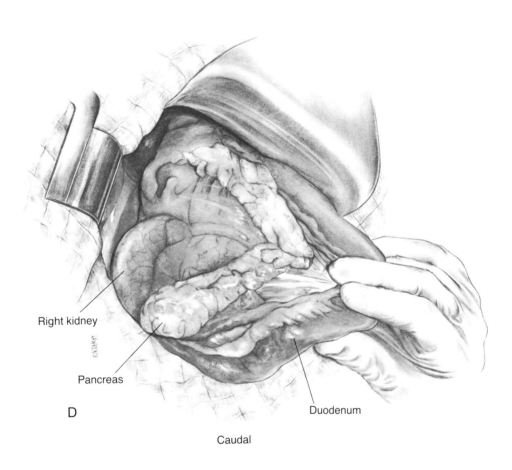

Right kidney

Pancreas

Duodenum

D

Caudal

Approach to the Adrenal Glands *continued*

DESCRIPTION OF THE PROCEDURE *continued*

E. The right lateral and caudate lobes of the liver are retracted cranially, exposing the cranial aspect of the right adrenal gland, which is visualized on the dorsolateral aspect of the caudal vena cava. The remainder of the gland is covered by the caudal vena cava and the retroperitoneal fat.

F. A combination of blunt and sharp dissection of surrounding fatty tissue and gentle medial retraction of the caudal vena cava is used to fully expose the gland. Care is taken during dissection to avoid damage to the caudal vena cava or to the caudally located renal artery and vein.

CLOSURE

The abdomen is closed as described in Approach to the Abdomen by Cranioventral Midline Celiotomy (see p 168).

COMMENT

The use of vascular metal clips for hemostasis is advantageous because of the depth of the operative field.

Neoplasia involving the right adrenal gland may invade the caudal vena cava, making dissection and complete excision difficult.

Some surgeons prefer to approach adrenalectomy with paralumbar celiotomy (see p 178). The authors prefer a ventral midline approach, which allows complete examination of the abdomen and both adrenal glands through a single incision.

Plate 68

Approach to the Adrenal Glands *continued*

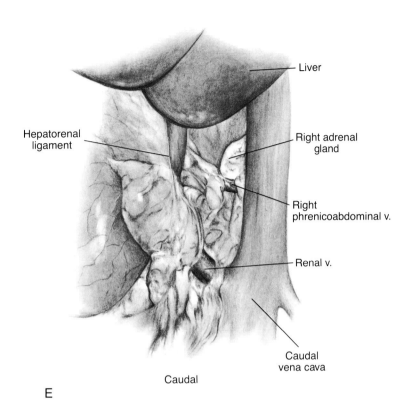

Liver

Hepatorenal
ligament

Right adrenal
gland

Right
phrenicoabdominal v.

Renal v.

Caudal
vena cava

Caudal

E

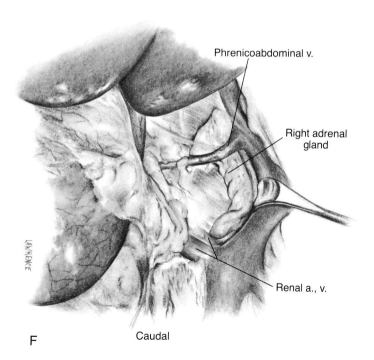

Phrenicoabdominal v.

Right adrenal
gland

Renal a., v.

Caudal

F

Approach to the Kidneys

INDICATIONS

Nephrectomy, nephrotomy, biopsy, and exploration of the urinary tract.

DESCRIPTION OF THE PROCEDURE

A. The patient is positioned in dorsal recumbency, and the abdomen is approached by cranioventral midline celiotomy (see p 166). Moistened laparotomy pads are placed to protect the abdominal wall, and self-retaining retractors are used to maintain visualization of the abdominal cavity. Ventromedial retraction of the duodenum and the mesoduodenum is used to pack abdominal viscera to the left, exposing the right kidney and the retroperitoneal space.

B. The descending colon and the mesocolon are retracted ventromedially, packing off viscera to the right, exposing the left kidney and the retroperitoneal space.

Plate 69

Approach to the Kidneys

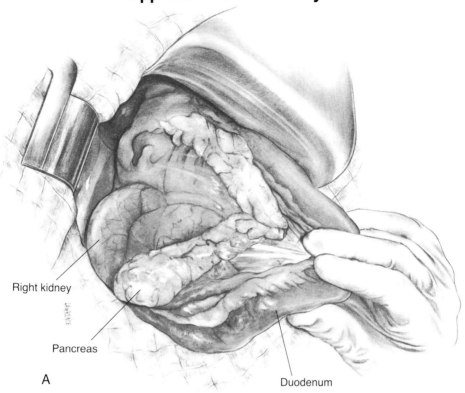

Right kidney

Pancreas

A

Caudal

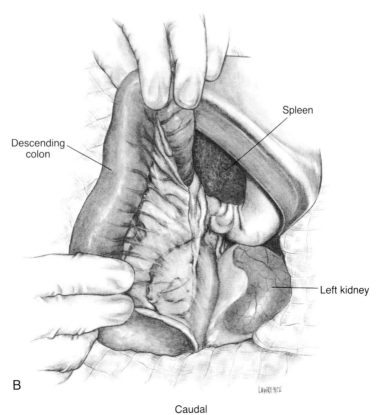

Descending
colon

Spleen

Duodenum

Left kidney

B

Caudal

Approach to the Kidneys *continued*

DESCRIPTION OF THE PROCEDURE *continued*

C. Nephrectomy is initiated by blunt and sharp dissection to free the kidney of peritoneal attachments and the renal capsule. The cranial pole of the right kidney is embedded in the fossa of the caudate lobe of the liver. The hepatorenal ligament may inhibit renal mobilization and is incised for nephrectomy if necessary. The renal artery is located craniodorsal and the vein caudoventral at the renal hilus. These vessels are ligated separately with nonabsorbable suture. The ureter leaves the renal pelvis and runs caudally in the retroperitoneal space to the urinary bladder. Ligation and division of the ureter are completed close to the urinary bladder.

D. Nephrotomy is performed for renal urolith removal. Temporary occlusion of the renal blood supply is achieved by vascular clamps or by digital compression using the index and middle fingers. Closure of the nephrotomy is initiated by holding the divided renal parenchyma together until fibrin and blood clot formation is sufficient to maintain apposition. A continuous pattern of synthetic absorbable suture is then placed in the renal capsule.

CLOSURE

The abdomen is closed as described in Approach to the Abdomen by Cranioventral Midline Celiotomy (see p 168).

COMMENTS

Excretory urography should be performed prior to nephrectomy or nephrotomy.

Variations in renal vascular anatomy are common (arterial branching), necessitating careful dissection of the vasculature during nephrectomy. In cases requiring nephrectomy, chronic disease or neoplasia may distort or destroy normal anatomy.

Prior to nephrotomy or nephrectomy, the contralateral kidney should be palpated and/ or examined for disease.

Bilateral nephrotomy at the same surgery is not recommended because of the decrease in renal function caused by incision.

All uroliths should be cultured and submitted for quantitative analysis.

Plate 69

Approach to the Kidneys *continued*

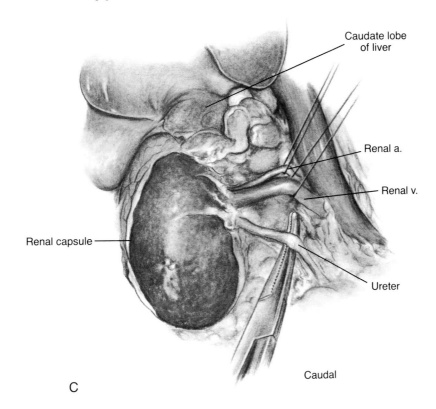

Caudate lobe of liver

Renal a.

Renal v.

Renal capsule

Ureter

Caudal

C

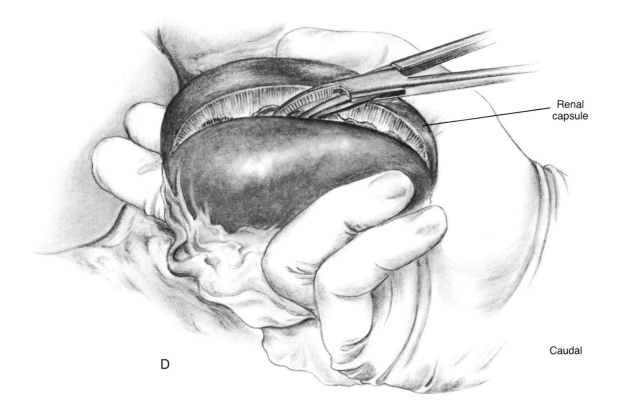

Renal capsule

Caudal

D

Approach to the Extravesicular Ureter

INDICATIONS

Management of ureteral trauma, ureteral obstruction, ectopic ureter, and iatrogenic ureteral injury.

DESCRIPTION OF THE PROCEDURE

A. The patient is positioned in dorsal recumbency, and the abdomen is approached by cranioventral or caudoventral midline celiotomy (see p 166, p 172, or p 174). Moistened laparotomy pads are placed to protect the abdominal wall, and self-retaining retractors are used to maintain visualization of the abdominal cavity. The left retroperitoneal space is exposed by ventromedial retraction of the colon, with the mesocolon used to pack viscera to the right. The right retroperitoneal space is exposed by ventromedial retraction on the duodenum, with the mesoduodenum used to pack viscera to the left. Each ureter leaves the renal pelvis and courses in the retroperitoneal space on the ventral surface of the psoas muscles.

Plate 70

Approach to the Extravesicular Ureter

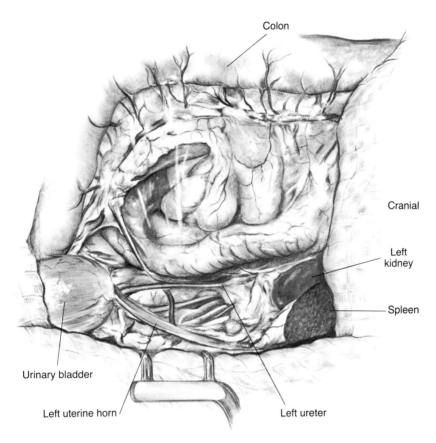

A

Approach to the Extravesicular Ureter *continued*

DESCRIPTION OF THE PROCEDURE *continued*

B. In the caudal abdomen, exposure of the ureter is enhanced by placement of a traction suture in the apex of the urinary bladder and caudoventral bladder retraction. The ureter leaves the retroperitoneal space in the caudal abdomen and passes dorsal to the ductus deferens in the male dog.

C. The ureters course through the lateral ligaments of the urinary bladder before entering the serosal surface on the dorsolateral aspect of the bladder just cranial to the bladder neck.

CLOSURE

The abdomen is closed as described in Approach to the Abdomen by Cranioventral Midline Celiotomy and Approach to the Abdomen by Caudoventral Midline Celiotomy (see p 168, p 172, or p 176).

COMMENTS

Excretory urography is valuable in determining the anatomic location of ureteral pathology.

In the female, the ureter is associated with the broad ligament of the uterus before reaching the lateral ligaments. Iatrogenic ureteral injury may occur during ovariohysterectomy close to the kidney or where the ureter leaves the retroperitoneal space caudally.

During exploratory cystotomy, it is often valuable to catheterize the ureters via the ureteral orifice located at the trigone. A ventral cystotomy is performed as demonstrated in Approach to the Urinary Bladder and the Intravesicular Ureter, Fig. **B** (see p 241). The ureter is catheterized with a no. 3 soft rubber or polyvinyl catheter.

Plate 70

Approach to the Extravesicular Ureter *continued*

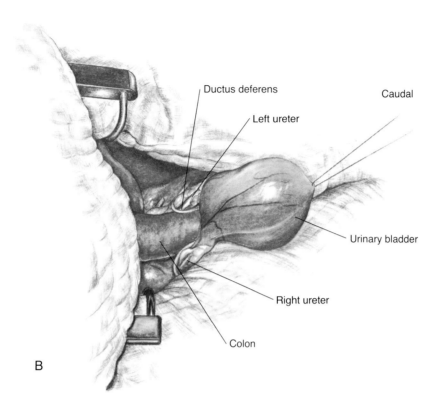

Ductus deferens

Left ureter

Caudal

Urinary bladder

Right ureter

Colon

B

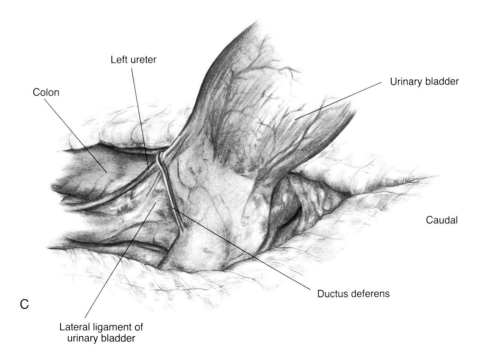

Left ureter

Colon

Urinary bladder

Caudal

Ductus deferens

Lateral ligament of
urinary bladder

C

Approach to the Urinary Bladder and the Intravesicular Ureter

INDICATIONS

Cystotomy for removal of cystic calculi, examination and catheterization of ureters, correction of intramural ectopic ureter, implantation of the ureter following renal transplantation or traumatic severance, and partial cystectomy for neoplasia.

DESCRIPTION OF THE PROCEDURE

A. The patient is positioned in dorsal recumbency, and the abdomen is approached by caudoventral midline celiotomy, with specifics of the technique depending on the sex of the patient (see p 172 or p 174). The urinary bladder is located in the caudal abdomen or pelvic inlet.

B. A stay suture is placed in the cranial aspect of the bladder to facilitate exteriorization of the bladder from the abdomen. Moistened laparotomy pads are used to isolate the bladder from the abdomen. Cystocentesis is performed to empty the bladder, and a stab incision is made in an avascular area of the ventral bladder wall. Stay sutures are placed lateral to the incision to allow complete inspection of the bladder. The ureters open at the trigone of the bladder by means of two slit-like openings on the dorsolateral wall.

Plate 71

Approach to the Urinary Bladder and the Intravesicular Ureter

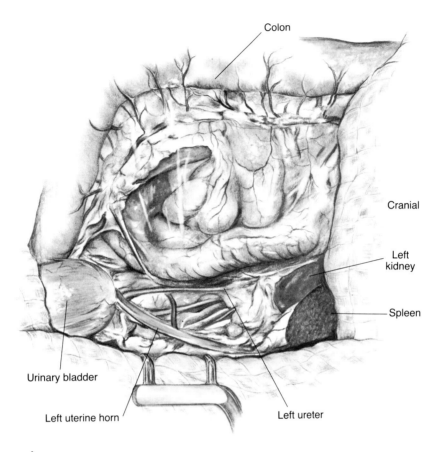

Colon

Cranial

Left kidney

Spleen

Urinary bladder

Left uterine horn

Left ureter

A

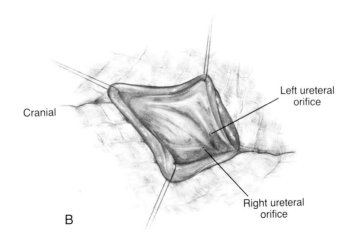

Cranial

Left ureteral orifice

Right ureteral orifice

B

Approach to the Urinary Bladder and the Intravesicular Ureter *continued*

DESCRIPTION OF THE PROCEDURE *continued*

C. The normal ureteral orifice may be catheterized with a no. 3 urinary catheter. In patients with ureteral ectopia, there is an absence or abnormal location of the intravesicular orifice despite a normal intramural location of the ureter(s). The ectopic ureter may be visualized as a tubular bulge below the ureteral mucosa. A no. 15 scalpel blade is used to incise the bladder mucosa and the ureteral wall. The edges of the ureteral incision are sutured to the bladder mucosa with small, absorbable suture (inset). The distal portion of the ectopic ureter is ligated to prevent further urine flow.

D. Implantation of a ureter during transplantation or following severance is performed by drawing the affected ureter by stay suture through a full-thickness stab incision in the bladder wall. The end of the ureter is excised, spatulated, and sutured to the bladder mucosa with small absorbable suture (inset). A catheter is used during suturing to ensure ureteral patency.

CLOSURE

The urinary bladder is closed with absorbable suture in a two-layer continuous inverting pattern. Suture should not penetrate the bladder lumen. The abdomen is closed as described in Approach to the Abdomen by Caudoventral Midline Celiotomy (see p 172 or p 176).

COMMENTS

Bladder wall closure is modified depending on bladder size and wall thickness. Cystotomy for calculi removal is made in a convenient hypovascular area of the bladder. Cystotomy for trigone exploration and ureteral catheterization is performed ventrally.

All calculi are submitted for quantitative analysis.

Care is taken during cystotomy or partial cystectomy to avoid damage to ureteral orifices in the trigone area.

Plate 71

Approach to the Urinary Bladder and the Intravesicular Ureter *continued*

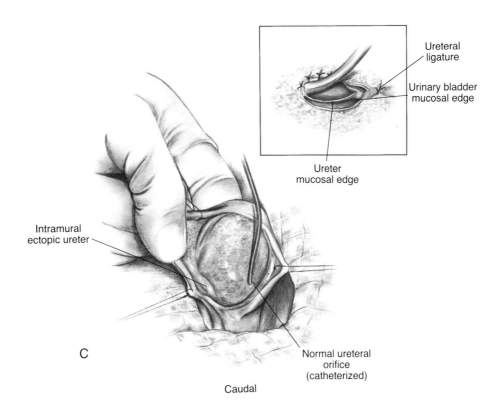

Ureteral ligature

Urinary bladder mucosal edge

Ureter mucosal edge

Intramural ectopic ureter

Normal ureteral orifice (catheterized)

C

Caudal

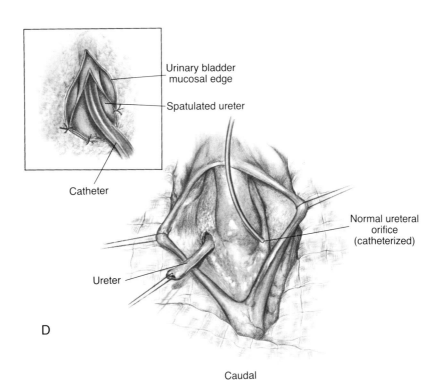

Urinary bladder mucosal edge

Spatulated ureter

Catheter

Normal ureteral orifice (catheterized)

Ureter

D

Caudal

Approach to the Uterus and the Ovary

INDICATIONS

Elective ovariohysterectomy, ovariohysterectomy for uterine disease, and cesarean section.

DESCRIPTION OF THE PROCEDURE

A. The patient is positioned in dorsal recumbency, and the abdomen is approached by caudoventral midline celiotomy (see p 172). The skin incision is shortened for elective ovariohysterectomy. In the normal animal, the right or left uterine horn is located by means of an ovariohysterectomy hook or an index finger. The uterine horn is followed cranially to the ovary, which is located just caudal to the kidney. The canine ovary is located within the ovarian bursa and is obscured by fat. The proper ligament of the ovary is located between the uterine horn and the ovarian bursa. A clamp is placed on this structure to facilitate placing traction on the ovary. The suspensory ligament extends between the ventral ovary and the twelfth or thirteenth rib and is stretched or torn prior to ligation of the ovarian vascular pedicle. The ovarian artery arises from the aorta and extends through the mesovarium to the ovary.

B. The broad ligament (mesometrium) is torn or severed to assist in exteriorization of the uterine horns and body. If the broad ligament is vascular, it should be ligated prior to being cut. The uterine arteries and veins supply the caudal uterus and are ligated just cranial to the cervix by mass ligation with the uterus. Alternatively, uterine vasculature may be individually ligated.

C. Ovariohysterectomy of the diseased uterus is similar to that performed on the normal uterus, but the skin incision is larger. If the patient is pregnant or the uterus is diseased, the uterine horns are distended and may fill the abdominal cavity, necessitating care on abdominal entry to avoid injury to the uterus or to other abdominal viscera.

Plate 72

Approach to the Uterus and the Ovary

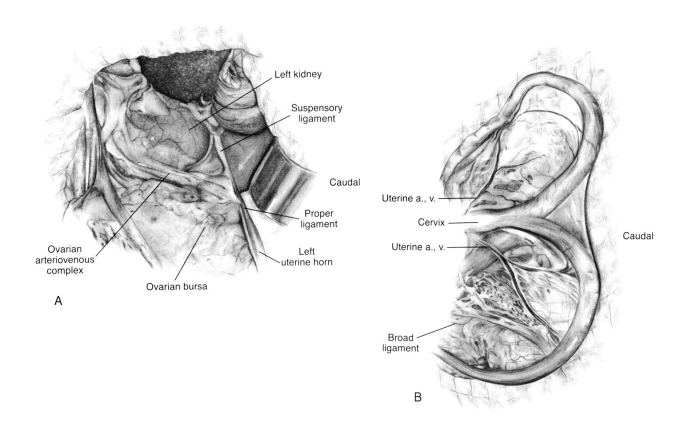

A

Left kidney

Suspensory ligament

Caudal

Proper ligament

Left uterine horn

Ovarian arteriovenous complex

Ovarian bursa

B

Uterine a., v.

Cervix

Uterine a., v.

Caudal

Broad ligament

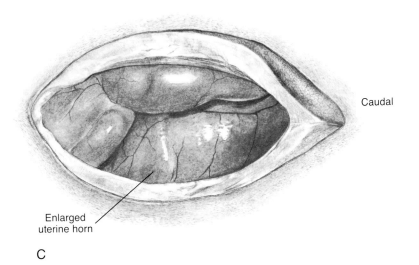

C

Caudal

Enlarged uterine horn

Approach to the Uterus and the Ovary *continued*

DESCRIPTION OF THE PROCEDURE *continued*

D. Moistened laparotomy pads are used to pack off the pregnant or diseased uterus. For cesarean section, a longitudinal incision is made in the uterine body of sufficient length to allow removal of the fetuses. Each uterine horn and the uterine body are carefully palpated to ensure extraction of all fetuses.

E. Fetal membranes are removed prior to closure of the uterine incision. Uterine involution begins immediately after fetal removal. The uterus is closed with a simple continuous pattern and oversewn with synthetic absorbable suture in an interrupted Lembert pattern.

CLOSURE

The abdomen is closed as described in Approach to the Abdomen by Caudoventral Midline Celiotomy in the Female Dog (see p 172).

COMMENTS

The urinary bladder is manually expressed prior to surgery.

Hemorrhage following ovariohysterectomy may be from ovarian, uterine, or broad ligament vasculature. The abdomen is checked for excessive hemorrhage prior to closure. If excessive hemorrhage occurs, each ovarian pedicle is located just caudal to the kidneys. The mesocolon on the left and the mesoduodenum on the right are used to retract abdominal viscera, assisting in exposure of each kidney and ovarian vascular pedicle. The uterine body pedicle is located between the urinary bladder and the colon; exposure is enhanced by caudoventral retraction of the bladder by stay suture.

Anatomy of the feline uterus and ovaries is similar. Exposure of the feline ovary and vascular pedicle is simplified by the lack of intraabdominal fat and the ease of exteriorization of the pedicle; thus, the skin incision may be made beginning 2 to 3 cm caudal to the umbilicus.

Elective ovariohysterectomy or ovariectomy is performed by a paralumbar approach in the United Kingdom. The authors do not have experience with ovariohysterectomy performed by this approach.

Plate 72

Approach to the Uterus and the Ovary *continued*

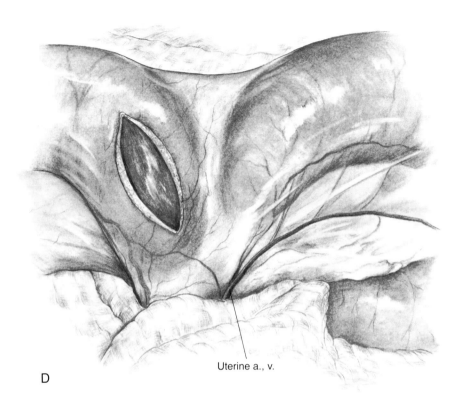

Uterine a., v.

D

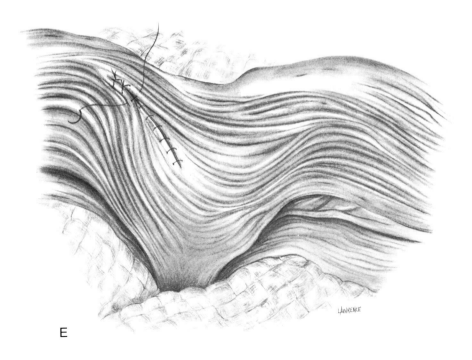

E

Approach to the Prostate

INDICATIONS

Open biopsy, prostatectomy, and drainage procedures for prostatic abscess and para-prostatic cysts.

DESCRIPTION OF THE PROCEDURE

A. The patient is positioned in dorsal recumbency, and the limbs are secured to the operating table. The abdominal cavity is approached by caudoventral midline celiotomy (see p 174).

B. The abdominal cavity is entered, and the urinary bladder is identified. A stay suture is placed in the apex of the urinary bladder to facilitate atraumatic tissue handling. Moistened laparotomy pads are placed to isolate the surgical field and to protect abdominal viscera. The prostate surrounds the proximal urethra caudal to the bladder neck and is covered by abundant periprostatic fat.

C. A polyvinyl or soft rubber urinary catheter is placed to aid in the identification of the urethra. Blunt dissection of surrounding fat exposes the prostate, which may be biopsied by sharp incision or needle device. If inflammatory, cystic, or neoplastic disease results in significant prostatomegaly, the prostate is readily apparent. If prostatectomy is to be performed (see Comments), multiple branches of the prostatic artery are isolated and ligated close to the dorsolateral aspect of the gland. Transection of the urethra is performed close to the gland cranially and caudally, and anastomosis of the urethra is performed over a catheter.

CLOSURE

A single interrupted suture of absorbable material may be necessary for hemostasis at prostatic biopsy sites. The abdomen is closed as described in Approach to the Abdomen by Caudoventral Midline Celiotomy in the Male Dog (see p 176).

COMMENTS

Ancillary surgical approaches for treatment of prostatic disease include castration and drainage techniques utilizing soft rubber drains for abscesses or marsupialization of paraprostatic cysts. Some cysts may be excised entirely from prostatic parenchyma. Castration should be performed for hyperplastic, inflammatory, or cystic disease.

The authors believe that prostatectomy is rarely indicated because of the high rate of postoperative urinary incontinence in dogs with prostatic disease.

Multiple biopsy samples may be indicated because several disease processes may be present concurrently. Aerobic and anaerobic bacterial cultures are routinely performed from biopsy sites or tissue samples.

Plate 73
Approach to the Prostate

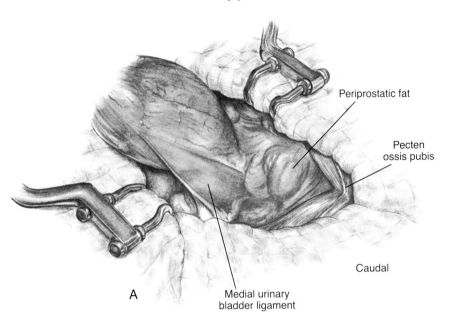

Periprostatic fat

Pecten
ossis pubis

Caudal

A

Medial urinary
bladder ligament

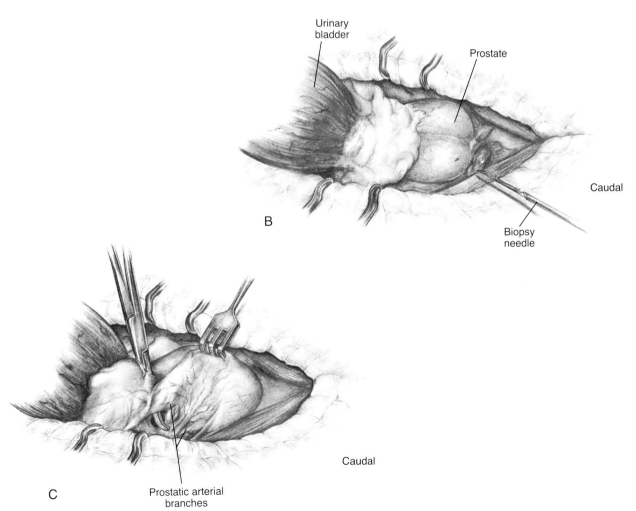

Urinary
bladder

Prostate

Caudal

B

Biopsy
needle

Caudal

C

Prostatic arterial
branches

Approach to the Medial Iliac Lymph Nodes

INDICATIONS

Incisional or excisional biopsy of the medial iliac lymph nodes to diagnose and/or stage neoplastic and inflammatory disease.

DESCRIPTION OF THE PROCEDURE

A. The patient is positioned in dorsal recumbency and the abdomen is approached by caudoventral midline celiotomy (see p 172 or p 174). Moistened laparotomy pads are placed to protect the abdominal wall, and self-retaining retractors are used to maintain visualization of the caudal abdominal cavity. The small intestine is retracted medially using the colon and the mesocolon and is protected with moistened laparotomy pads. The aorta and the caudal vena cava lie in the furrow that is formed by the psoas muscles on the ventral surface of the lumbar vertebrae.

Plate 74
Approach to the Medial Iliac Lymph Nodes

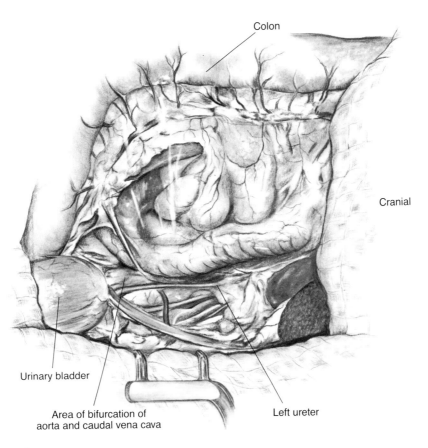

Colon

Cranial

Urinary bladder

Area of bifurcation of
aorta and caudal vena cava

Left ureter

A

Approach to the Medial Iliac Lymph Nodes *continued*

DESCRIPTION OF THE PROCEDURE *continued*

B. The medial iliac lymph nodes lie on each side of the aorta between the deep circumflex iliac and external iliac arteries and veins. Depending on body condition, the lymph nodes are surrounded by varying amounts of fatty tissue.

C. A combination of blunt and sharp dissection is used to expose and excise the lymph node. Care is taken to avoid disruption of the major arterial and venous structures, which lie close to the lymph node.

CLOSURE

The abdomen is closed as described in Approach to the Abdomen by Caudoventral Midline Celiotomy (see p 172 or p 176).

COMMENTS

The medial iliac lymph nodes are commonly known as sublumbar lymph nodes, a term that refers to their location ventral to the bodies of the fifth and sixth lumbar vertebrae.

Plate 74

Approach to the Medial Iliac Lymph Nodes *continued*

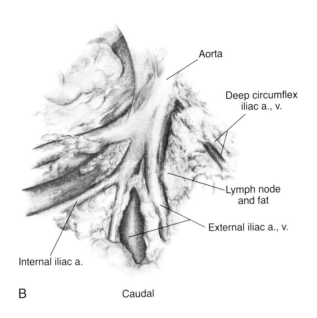

Aorta

Deep circumflex
iliac a., v.

Lymph node
and fat

External iliac a., v.

Internal iliac a.

B   Caudal

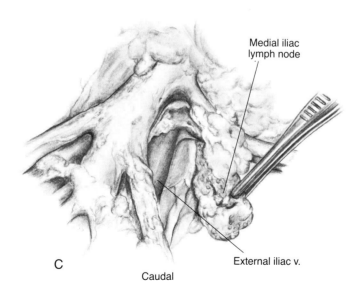

Medial iliac
lymph node

External iliac v.

C   Caudal

Extraabdominal Urogenital Surgery

Topographic Penile and Urethral Anatomy: Canine

Urethral anatomy in cross-section referred to in discussions of approaches to the perineal, scrotal, prescrotal, and distal urethra in the canine (see further on in this chapter).

I. Perineal
   A. Urethra
   B. Corpus spongiosum penis
   C. Bulb of penis
   D. Bulbospongiosus muscle
   E. Retractor penis muscle
II. Scrotal
   A. Ischiocavernosus muscle
   B. Crus of corpus cavernosum
   C. Corpus spongiosum penis
   D. Urethra
   E. Bulbospongiosus muscle
   F. Retractor penis muscle
III. Prescrotal
   A. Corpus cavernosum
   B. Tunica albuginea
   C. Urethra
   D. Corpus spongiosum penis
   E. Retractor penis muscle
IV. Midbody
   A. Bulbus glandis
   B. Os penis
   C. Urethra
   D. Anastomosis of bulbus glandis and corpus spongiosum penis
V. Distal
   A. Pars longa glandis
   B. Os penis
   C. Urethra
   D. Corpus spongiosum penis

Based on Christensen GC: The urogenital apparatus. In *Evans HE, and Christensen GC (eds): Miller's Anatomy of the Dog. Philadelphia, WB Saunders, 1979, p 568.*

Plate 75

Topographic Penile and Urethral Anatomy: Canine

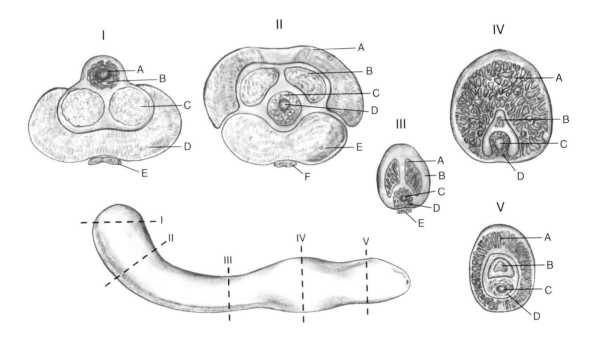

Approach to the Perineal Urethra: Canine

INDICATIONS

Obstruction of the urethra by calculi, stricture, or neoplasia and traumatic disruption of the urethra between the scrotum and the ischial arch.

DESCRIPTION OF THE PROCEDURE

A. A no. 5 or no. 8 urethral catheter is placed, and the patient is positioned in ventral recumbency. A purse-string suture is placed in the anus, and the tail is positioned dorsally and maintained with tape. A midline perineal skin incision is centered between the anus and the scrotum.

B. Subcutaneous tissues are incised to the level of the retractor penis muscle, which is elevated and retracted laterally, exposing the bulbospongiosus muscles. The bulbospongiosus muscles are divided on midline. The corpus spongiosum penis is incised over the urinary catheter to expose the urethral lumen.

Plate 76
Approach to the Perineal Urethra: Canine

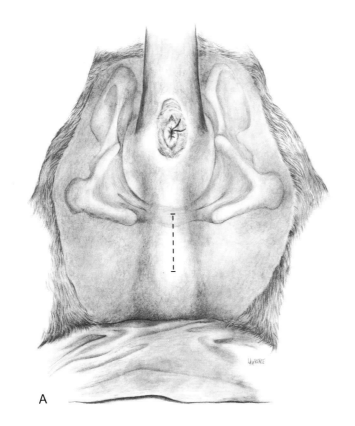

A

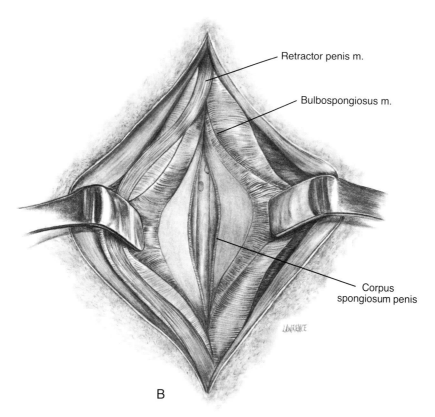

Retractor penis m.

Bulbospongiosus m.

Corpus
spongiosum penis

B

Approach to the Perineal Urethra: Canine *continued*

DESCRIPTION OF THE PROCEDURE *continued*

C. Following urethrotomy for calculi, the perineal urethra is meticulously closed with 5-0 synthetic absorbable suture in a simple interrupted pattern. Permanent urethrostomy may be performed by suturing the urethral mucosa to the skin dorsally at the 11-, 12-, and 1-o'clock positions (inset) with interrupted sutures of 4-0 nylon or polypropylene.

CLOSURE

If urethral closure is performed, the subcutaneous tissues are apposed with absorbable suture in a continuous or interrupted pattern. The skin is closed with nonabsorbable suture in a simple interrupted pattern.

COMMENTS

Scrotal urethrostomy is the preferred surgical technique for permanent urethrostomy.

The perineal urethra is more difficult to approach because of its distance from the skin and because of the presence of the bulbospongiosus muscles. A potential complication of perineal urethrostomy in the dog is urine scalding of the perineum or scrotum.

Postoperative hemorrhage from the corpus spongiosum penis is minimized by meticulous suturing of the urethral mucosa. Intermittent dripping of blood from the urethrostomy site, hematuria, or both are common for the first 3 postoperative days.

The dog should be monitored long-term for bacterial urinary tract infection.

Plate 76

Approach to the Perineal Urethra: Canine *continued*

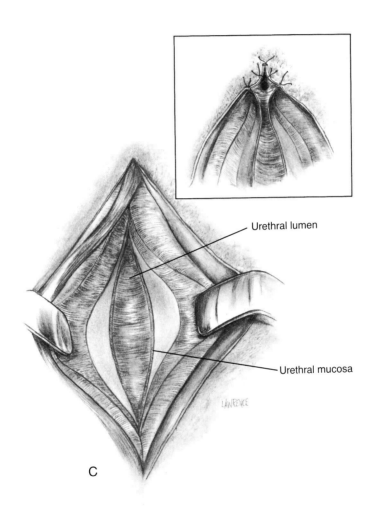

Urethral lumen

Urethral mucosa

C

Approach to the Scrotal Urethra: Canine

INDICATIONS

Permanent scrotal urethrostomy and amputation of the prepuce and the penis.

DESCRIPTION OF THE PROCEDURE

A. The patient is positioned in dorsal recumbency with the rear limbs in the frog-leg position. An elliptical skin incision is made to encompass the scrotum and the testes at the scrotal base. The scrotum is completely excised (see p 274).

B. Castration is performed by the open or closed method (see p 275) and the scrotal urethra is exposed by elevation of the retractor penis muscle. A no. 5 or no. 8 urinary catheter is passed to aid in identification of the urethral lumen.

C. The urethral lumen is entered by incision over the catheter with a scalpel. The urethral incision is approximately 2.5 to 3.0 cm long and extends caudally to where the urethra begins to curve dorsally.

CLOSURE

The surgeon begins urethrostomy by suturing the urethral mucosa to the skin at the cranial and caudal aspects of the incision with 3-0 or 4-0 nylon or polypropylene in a simple interrupted pattern (inset). The remainder of the urethral mucosa is sutured to the skin with an interrupted or continuous pattern. Skin that is not sutured to the urethra is closed with nonabsorbable suture.

COMMENTS

Scrotal urethrostomy creates permanent urinary diversion and is most commonly indicated in dogs that chronically form urinary calculi, which may cause urethral obstruction at the base of the os penis. Stricture of the prescrotal urethra at a previous urethrotomy site and penile-preputial excision for neoplastic disease also are indications for the procedure.

Postoperative hemorrhage from incised corpus spongiosum penis is minimized by meticulous suturing of the urethral mucosa. Intermittent dripping of blood from the incision, hematuria, or both are common for the first 3 postoperative days.

The dog should be monitored long-term for bacterial urinary tract infection.

Plate 77

Approach to the Scrotal Urethra: Canine

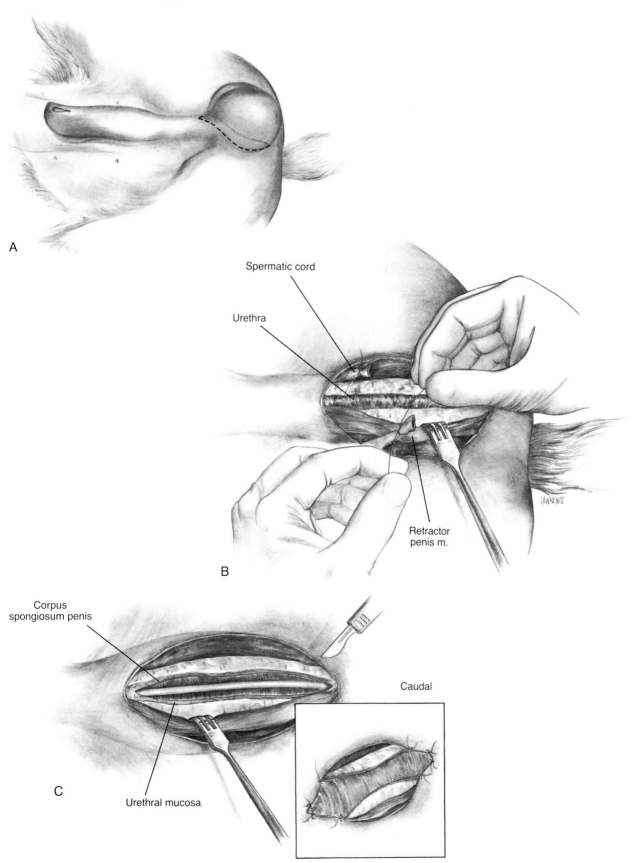

A

Spermatic cord

Urethra

Retractor
penis m.

B

Corpus
spongiosum penis

Caudal

Urethral mucosa

C

Approach to the Prescrotal Urethra: Canine

INDICATIONS

Urethrotomy for urethral calculi removal and permanent urethrostomy for distal urethral obstruction.

DESCRIPTION OF THE PROCEDURE

A. The patient is placed in dorsal recumbency. A skin incision is made from the base of the os penis to the base of the scrotum.

B. Subcutaneous tissue is incised, and the retractor penis muscle is isolated and retracted. A polyvinyl or soft rubber urinary catheter is passed to the level of the obstruction, and the urethra is elevated from the incision.

Plate 78

Approach to the Prescrotal Urethra: Canine

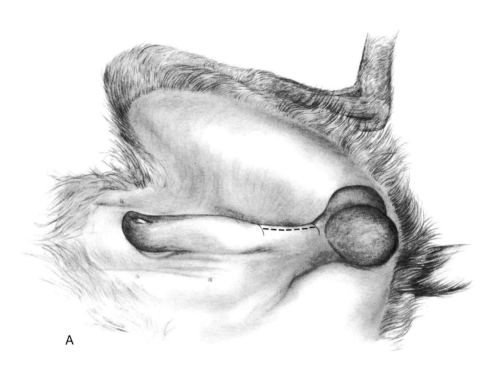

A

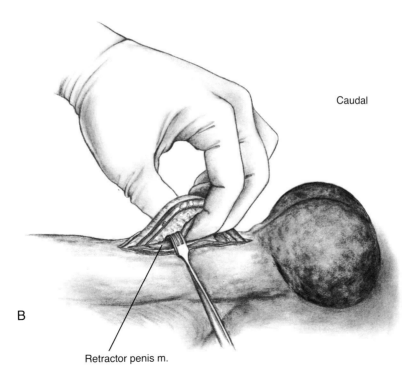

Caudal

B

Retractor penis m.

Approach to the Prescrotal Urethra: Canine *continued*

DESCRIPTION OF THE PROCEDURE *continued*

C. The urethral lumen is entered directly on midline by sharp incision over the calculi or the urinary catheter with a no. 15 scalpel blade. The incision is extended with iris scissors. Following calculi removal, the urethra is flushed copiously with saline, and the catheter is passed to the bladder to ensure urethral patency.

CLOSURE

The urethral mucosa is meticulously closed with 5-0 synthetic absorbable suture on a tapered needle (inset). A continuous or interrupted intradermal-subcutaneous tissue closure performed with absorbable suture provides good skin apposition and precludes the need for skin sutures, which may contribute to self-trauma in this area.

COMMENTS

The pressure from digital elevation of the urethra from the incision decreases hemorrhage from the incised corpus spongiosum penis.

Suture closure of the urethra is optional. If the urethral mucosa is unhealthy or if minimizing operative time is necessary because of uremia, the urethra and the surgical wound may heal by second intention. Closure of the urethra minimizes hemorrhage in the postoperative period.

Cystotomy may be necessary to remove concurrent bladder calculi.

All calculi removed should be submitted for quantitative analysis.

The prescrotal urethra may be selected for permanent urethrostomy if castration cannot be performed. The urethra is wider and more superficial caudally at the scrotal level, making scrotal urethrostomy the preferred technique for permanent urethrostomy, as illustrated in Approach to the Scrotal Urethra (see p 262).

Plate 78

Approach to the Prescrotal Urethra: Canine *continued*

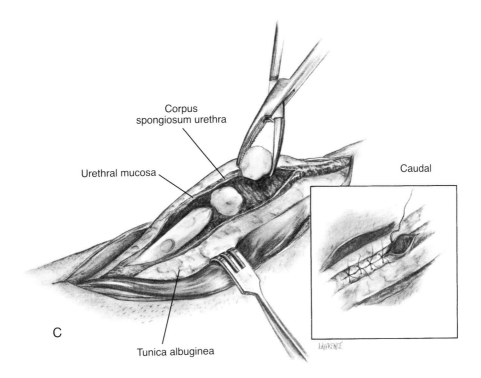

Corpus
spongiosum urethra

Urethral mucosa

Tunica albuginea

Caudal

C

Approach to the Distal Penile Urethra: Canine

INDICATIONS

Distal urethral injury or prolapse, penile neoplasia, and vascular compromise of the distal penis.

DESCRIPTION OF THE PROCEDURE

A. The patient is positioned in dorsal recumbency. The ventral abdomen and the preputial cavity are prepared for surgery, and the urethra is catheterized. The prepuce is retracted caudally, and a rubber tourniquet is placed around the penis caudally. A circumferential incision is made through the pars longa glandis, illustrated in Topographic Penile and Urethral Anatomy: Canine (p 256).

B. The urethra is dissected from the groove in the os penis, and partial ostectomy of the os penis is performed using bone cutters or rongeurs. The urethra is transected distal to the penile amputation site to provide sufficient urethral mucosa to cover the amputation site. A longitudinal incision is made in the remaining urethra to facilitate urethral and penile mucosal apposition. The tourniquet may be loosened to identify and ligate vessels in the erectile tissue; however, hemorrhage tends to be diffuse and ligation difficult.

CLOSURE

The urethral mucosa is sutured to the penile mucosa of the distal penile amputation site with synthetic absorbable suture in a simple interrupted pattern.

COMMENTS

Intermittent hemorrhage from the incised corpus spongiosum penis is common during the first 3 postoperative days.

Plate 79

Approach to the Distal Penile Urethra: Canine

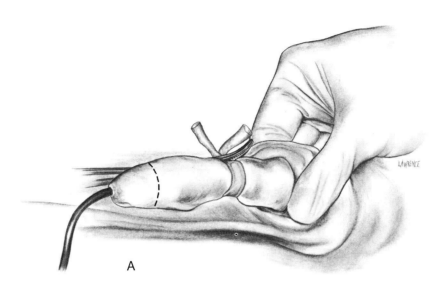

A

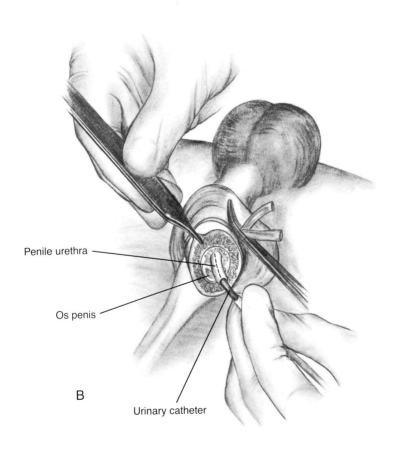

Penile urethra

Os penis

B

Urinary catheter

Approach to the Penis: Canine

INDICATIONS

Penile amputation for neoplasia, congenital deformity, vascular compromise, and traumatic injury causing permanent dysfunction.

DESCRIPTION OF THE PROCEDURE

A. The patient is positioned in dorsal recumbency. Following scrotal ablation and castration, described in Approach to the Scrotum: Canine (see p 274), the ventral midline skin incision is extended to the cranial third of the prepuce. Subcutaneous tissues are dissected, and vascular supply to the penis is identified.

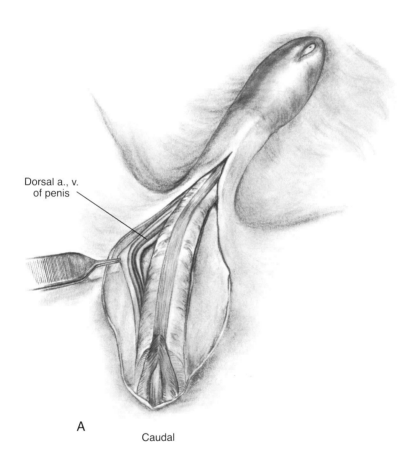

Plate 80

Approach to the Penis: Canine

Dorsal a., v. of penis

A

Caudal

Approach to the Penis: Canine *continued*

DESCRIPTION OF THE PROCEDURE *continued*

B. The dorsal artery and vein of the penis are ligated. Amputation includes resection of the retractor penis, the bulbospongiosus muscle, and the ischiocavernosus muscles at a location similar to part II of the illustration on p 256. The vascular corpus cavernosum and corpus spongiosum are divided in the same plane. A catheter placed in the urethra aids orientation during the amputation.

C. The distal segment of the amputated penis is retracted caudally. This maneuver delivers the submucosa of the parietal preputial mucosa into the operative field. The parietal mucosa is incised from inside-out at the level of the palpable distal penis. The mucosa is sutured with synthetic absorbable suture in a simple continuous pattern as the incision is made (inset).

CLOSURE

Soft latex drains are placed in the dorsal aspect of the wound and exited through periincisional stab wounds. Subcutaneous tissues are apposed with synthetic absorbable suture in a simple interrupted pattern. Skin is apposed with nonabsorbable suture in a simple interrupted pattern.

COMMENTS

This technique obviates amputation of the prepuce or incision of the entire ventral prepuce.

A circumferential absorbable suture may be placed around the distal end of the proximal segment of the amputated penis to provide hemostasis.

Penile amputation must be combined with either a scrotal or a perineal permanent urethrostomy. The urethra is ligated distal to the urethrostomy site.

Drains are placed to minimize fluid accumulation in dead space. They are removed 3 to 5 days after surgery.

Plate 80

Approach to the Penis: Canine *continued*

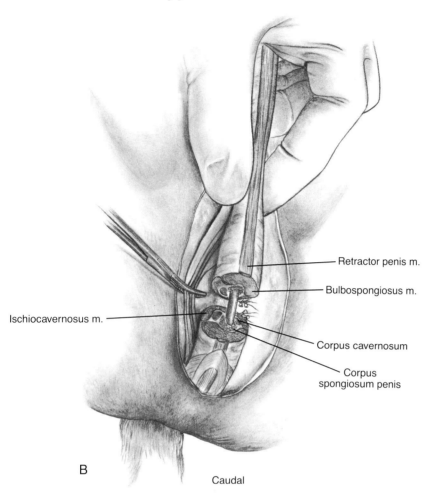

Retractor penis m.

Bulbospongiosus m.

Ischiocavernosus m.

Corpus cavernosum

Corpus spongiosum penis

B

Caudal

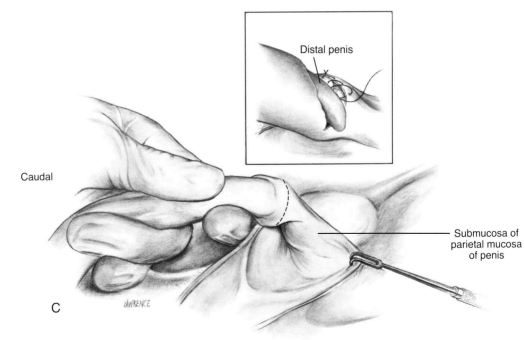

Distal penis

Caudal

Submucosa of parietal mucosa of penis

C

Approach to the Scrotum: Canine

INDICATIONS

Scrotal ablation for neoplasia and elective castration.

DESCRIPTION OF THE PROCEDURE

A. The patient is positioned in dorsal recumbency with the rear limbs in the frog-leg position. Slight traction is placed on the scrotum and the testes, and an elliptical skin incision is made 1 cm from the base of the scrotum at the body wall.

B. Traction is maintained on the scrotum and the testes while blunt dissection of subcutaneous tissue and fat facilitates exposure of the spermatic cords.

C. Castration is performed by the open or closed method, and the scrotum and the testicles are removed.

CLOSURE

An intradermal-subcutaneous tissue closure is performed with absorbable suture in an interrupted or continuous pattern. The skin is closed with nonabsorbable suture in a simple interrupted pattern.

COMMENTS

The skin incision is carefully placed. If the incision is made at the scrotal base–body wall junction, too much skin will be excised, resulting in excessive tension during closure. Cosmetic closure of the wound is difficult, and a dog-ear appearance is common. Wound contraction results in a satisfactory appearance. If a meticulous intradermal closure is performed, skin sutures may be omitted, which may reduce self-trauma.

Scrotal ablation and castration for elective neutering produce a pleasing cosmetic result in dogs with a pendulous scrotum.

The authors recommend open castration to minimize the risk of hemorrhage.

Plate 81
Approach to the Scrotum: Canine

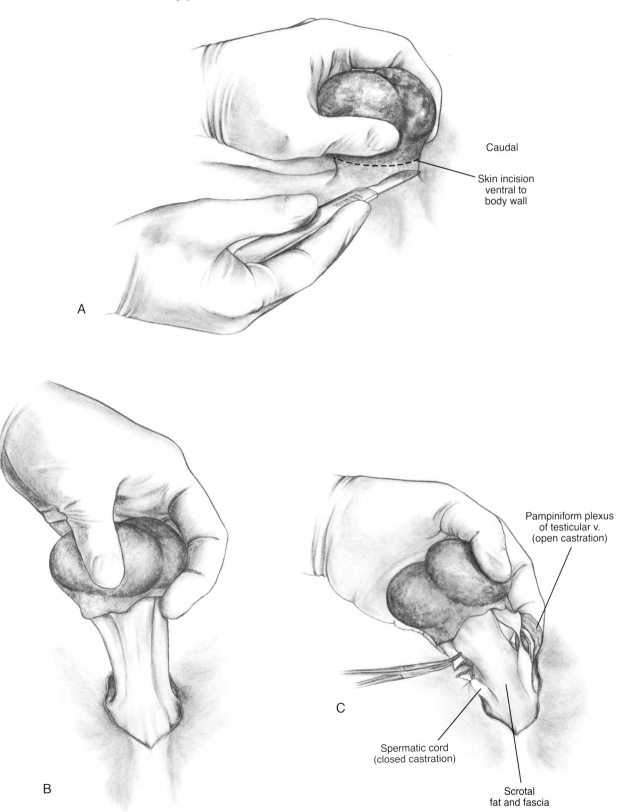

Caudal

Skin incision
ventral to
body wall

A

B

C

Pampiniform plexus
of testicular v.
(open castration)

Spermatic cord
(closed castration)

Scrotal
fat and fascia

Approach to the Testicles: Canine

INDICATIONS

Open biopsy and castration for elective neutering, testicular neoplasia, trauma, and torsion. Castration as adjunctive therapy for prostatic disease, perineal hernia, and perianal adenomas.

DESCRIPTION OF THE PROCEDURE

A. The patient is positioned in dorsal recumbency. A skin incision is made from the caudal base of the os penis to the cranial base of the scrotum.

B. The testis is pushed to the incision and exteriorized by incision of the subcutaneous tissue and the spermatic fascia over the testis. The parietal vaginal tunic is incised with a scalpel or scissors, and the testicle is expressed from the tunic. The tunica albuginea should be visualized but not incised.

Plate 82
Approach to the Testicles: Canine

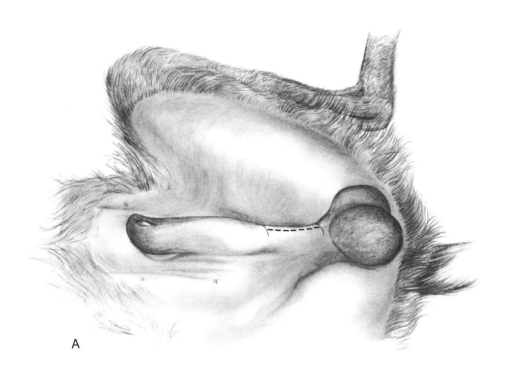

A

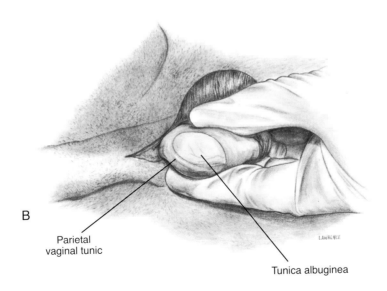

B

Parietal
vaginal tunic

Tunica albuginea

Approach to the Testicles: Canine *continued*

DESCRIPTION OF THE PROCEDURE *continued*

C. The tunic and the associated cremaster muscle have been manually avulsed with an instrument from the caudal aspect of the testis. The spermatic cord components are separated between the pampiniform plexus and the vas deferens. The testicular artery and the ductus deferens are isolated together, and the pampiniform plexus is isolated separately, with the three-clamp technique. The testes are removed following placement of two circumferential ligatures of absorbable suture.

CLOSURE

An intradermal-subcutaneous tissue closure is performed with fine synthetic absorbable suture. The skin is closed with nonabsorbable suture in a simple interrupted pattern.

COMMENTS

The tunic and the cremaster muscle may be avulsed or incised at their attachment to the testis (the ligament of the scrotum). If they are incised, the tunic should be ligated to prevent hemorrhage from a small accompanying vessel, which may cause scrotal hematoma.

In small dogs, the spermatic cord components may be safely mass ligated.

The authors recommend open castration to minimize the risk of hemorrhage. If closed castration is elected, fat and fascia surrounding each spermatic cord is reflected with a gauze sponge, and the spermatic cord is ligated by transfixation and with circumferential ligatures.

If a meticulous intradermal closure is performed, skin sutures can be omitted, which may reduce self-trauma.

Plate 82

Approach to the Testicles: Canine *continued*

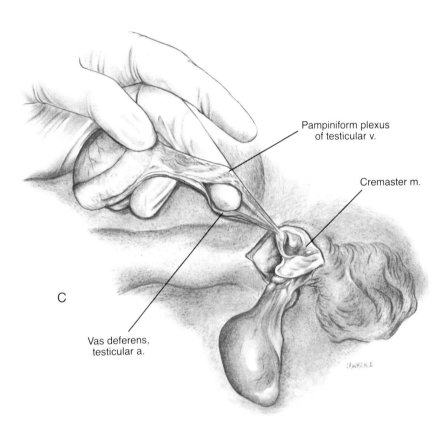

Pampiniform plexus
of testicular v.

Cremaster m.

C

Vas deferens,
testicular a.

Approach to the Vagina

INDICATIONS

Episiotomy for exploration of the vagina or the vestibule for congenital anomalies, neoplasia, and vaginal prolapse.

DESCRIPTION OF THE PROCEDURE

A. The patient is positioned in ventral recumbency, and the rear quarters are elevated with rolled towels or sandbags. A purse-string suture is placed in the anus. A skin incision is made extending from the dorsal vulvar commissure toward the anus.

B. The incision continues through the fascia, the constrictor vestibuli muscle, the vestibular bulb, and the vaginal mucosa. A urinary catheter is placed to protect and identify the urethra during excision of neoplastic or prolapsed tissue.

CLOSURE

The episiotomy incision is closed in three layers. Closure begins with a continuous pattern of absorbable suture in the vaginal mucosa. The muscular tissue and the submucosa are apposed with a continuous pattern of absorbable suture, and the skin is closed with nonabsorbable suture in simple interrupted pattern.

COMMENTS

A restraining collar may be used to prevent the patient from disrupting the suture line.

Based on a procedure of Blakely CL: The vulva. In Mayer K, Lacroix JV, and Hoskins HP (eds): Canine Surgery. Santa Barbara, CA, American Veterinary Publications, 1957, p 405.

Plate 83

Approach to the Vagina

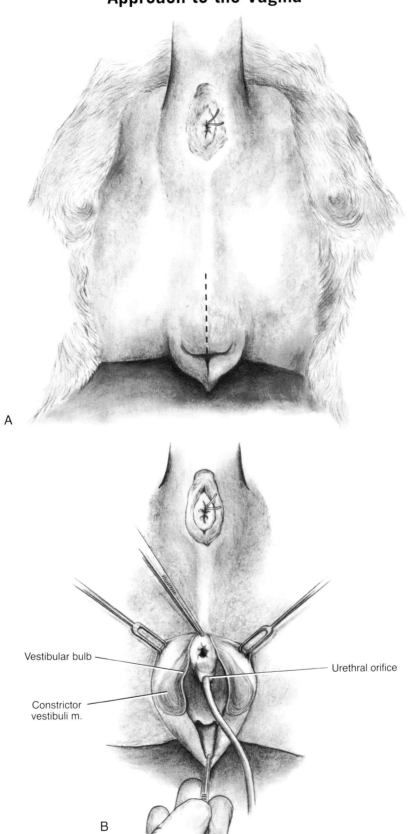

A

Vestibular bulb

Urethral orifice

Constrictor
vestibuli m.

B

Approach to the Mammary Glands

INDICATIONS

Lumpectomy, simple mammectomy, regional mastectomy, and complete mastectomy for neoplasia.

DESCRIPTION OF THE PROCEDURE

A. The patient is positioned in dorsal recumbency, with the rear limbs placed in the frog-leg position. An elliptical incision is made around the mammary glands to be excised. Subcutaneous tissues are sharply incised, and the body wall is exposed.

B. A plane of dissection is developed between the subcutaneous tissues and the external rectus abdominis muscle fascia for glands 3 to 5. For glands 1 and 2, dissection is performed between the pectoral musculature and the subcutaneous tissue. Inguinal gland excision necessitates removal of inguinal fat containing the inguinal lymph node. The caudal superficial epigastric artery and vein are ligated separately with synthetic absorbable suture as they emerge from the inguinal ring caudodorsal to the inguinal gland.

CLOSURE

Following simple, regional, or complete mastectomy, closure is initiated by placement of absorbable suture in a continuous or interrupted intradermal-subcutaneous tissue pattern. The skin is closed with nonabsorbable suture in a simple interrupted pattern.

COMMENTS

Care is taken to minimize dead space during closure by tacking subcutaneous tissues to the body wall.

Postoperative complications include wound dehiscence, seroma formation, and edema of the rear limbs. Rear limb edema caused by operative disruption of inguinal lymphatic drainage resolves with mild exercise and time.

Selection of the proper surgical procedure for mammary gland neoplasia is dictated by both the patient status and the nature and extent of the disease. Neoplastic tissue is widely excised, and generous normal tissue margins are desirable.

Neoplastic tissue and the excised lymph node are submitted for histologic examination.

Plate 84
Approach to the Mammary Glands

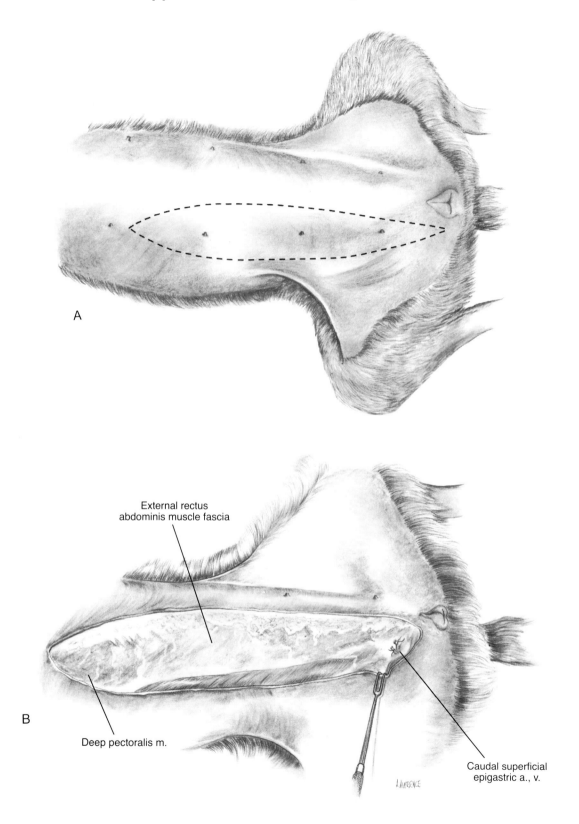

A

External rectus
abdominis muscle fascia

Deep pectoralis m.

Caudal superficial
epigastric a., v.

B

Approach to the Perineal Urethra: Feline

INDICATIONS

Urethral obstruction in male cats secondary to feline urologic syndrome; trauma of the penile urethra.

DESCRIPTION OF THE PROCEDURE

A. The patient is positioned in dorsal recumbency, and a purse-string suture is placed around the anus. An elliptical skin incision is made around the scrotum and the prepuce, and the cat is neutered if necessary. The prepuce and the scrotum are excised. Hemorrhage from the cranial and caudal scrotal arteries is controlled by cautery.

B. The penis is isolated and dissected from surrounding fatty tissue. The ischiocavernosus muscles are isolated bilaterally by blunt dissection, and they are transected close to their ischial attachments.

C. The penis is retracted dorsally, and the fibrous ventral penile ligament is transected with scissors. Blunt dissection is performed ventrally and laterally to completely free the pelvic urethra from its pelvic attachments.

Plate 85
Approach to the Perineal Urethra: Feline

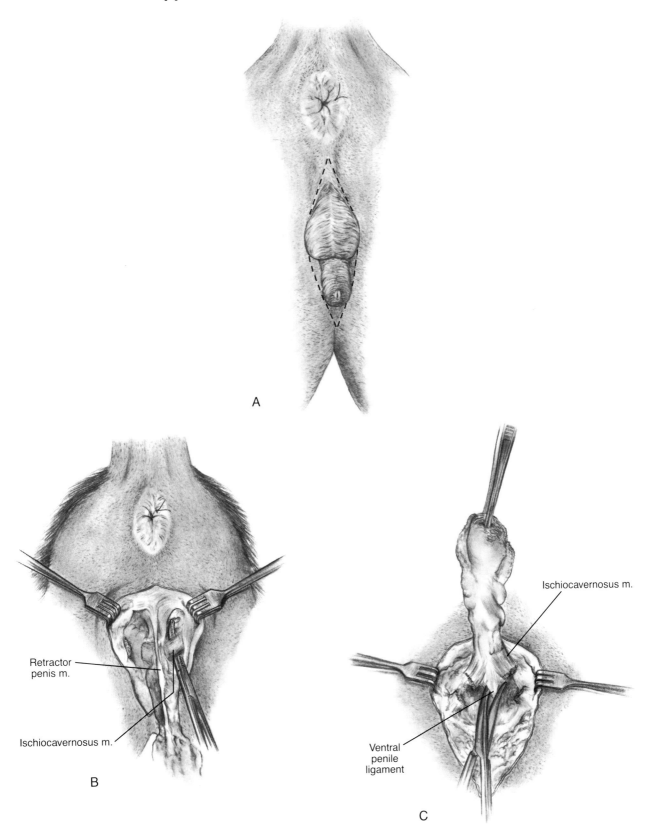

A

B

Retractor
penis m.

Ischiocavernosus m.

C

Ischiocavernosus m.

Ventral
penile
ligament

Approach to the Perineal Urethra: Feline *continued*

DESCRIPTION OF THE PROCEDURE *continued*

D. The retractor penis muscle is excised from the dorsal aspect of the urethra to the level of the bulbourethral glands. The penis is amputated, and the penile urethra is incised with iris scissors to the level of the bulbourethral glands. The glands are atrophied in cats that have been previously neutered and are just proximal to the ischiocavernosus muscle attachments. A through-and-through mattress suture is placed in the distal penile urethra to control hemorrhage from the incised corpus spongiosum penis.

CLOSURE

E. The surgeon begins urethrostomy by suturing the urethral mucosa to the skin dorsally with interrupted sutures of 4-0 nylon or polypropylene at the 11-, 12-, and 1-o'clock positions (inset). The remainder of the urethral mucosa is sutured to the skin in an interrupted or continuous pattern. The ventral portion of the skin incision is closed with nonabsorbable suture in an interrupted pattern, and the purse-string suture is removed from the anus.

COMMENTS

Hemorrhage from the ischiocavernosus muscles and the underlying penile crura is minimized by myotomy of the tendinous attachment to the ischium.

Dorsal dissection should be minimized to prevent damage to the rectum, the external anal sphincter muscle, and the pelvic nerves.

The urethra *must* be incised to the level of the bulbourethral glands to ensure that the pelvic urethra has been reached.

Meticulous suturing of the urethral mucosa to skin will minimize postoperative hemorrhage and stricture.

Indwelling urinary catheters are not recommended postoperatively. A restraining collar is used to prevent self-trauma. Shredded paper is used instead of litter until healing is complete.

The patient is sedated for suture removal to minimize trauma to the urethrostomy site.

Based on a procedure of Wilson GP, and Harrison JW: Perineal urethrostomy in cats. J Am Vet Med Assoc 159:1789, 1971.

Plate 85

Approach to the Perineal Urethra: Feline *continued*

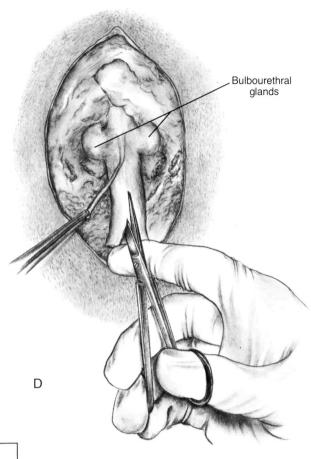

Bulbourethral
glands

D

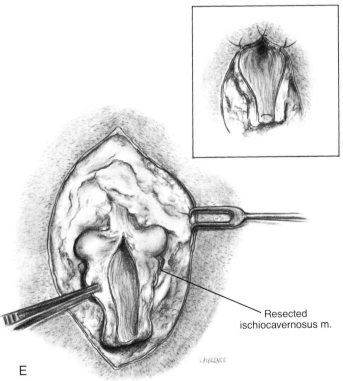

E

Resected
ischiocavernosus m.

Approach to the Prepubic Urethra: Feline

INDICATIONS

Neoplastic or inflammatory disease of the pelvic urethra, trauma to the pelvic urethra, and failed perineal urethrostomy.

DESCRIPTION OF THE PROCEDURE

A. The patient is positioned in dorsal recumbency, and all four limbs are secured to the operating table. A ventral midline skin incision is made beginning at the umbilicus cranially and extending to the level of the pecten ossis pubis caudally. (See p 173, Fig. **A.**) The abdominal cavity is entered, and the urinary bladder is identified. The urethra is isolated by blunt dissection of the abundant periurethral fatty tissue located between the bladder and the pecten ossis pubis.

B. A circumferential ligature of absorbable suture is placed around the caudal urethra as it enters the pelvic canal. The urethra is transected, and a stay suture is placed in the cranial urethra to facilitate atraumatic tissue handling. The urethra is freed of its dorsal attachments for a short distance to aid in exteriorization of the cranial urethral segment.

C. Stab incisions are made through the abdominal wall and skin lateral to the linea alba and skin incisions. The urethra is exteriorized ventrally and incised longitudinally (spatulated) with sharp iris scissors.

CLOSURE

Urethrostomy is performed by suturing the urethra to skin with 4-0 or 5-0 nylon or polypropylene (inset). The abdominal wall, the subcutaneous tissues, and the skin are closed separately.

COMMENTS

Excessive dissection of tissues of the dorsal periurethral area and the urinary bladder neck may result in urinary incontinence. The pecten ossis pubis may be osteotomized or removed with rongeurs to make available additional urethra to perform the procedure. This maneuver is rarely necessary.

Some surgeons exteriorize the urethra and locate the urethral stoma in the primary incision. Regardless of technique, excessive angulation (kinking) between the bladder neck and the urethra should be avoided.

One or two sutures may be placed between periurethral tissue and the external rectus abdominis muscle fascia to decrease tension on stomal sutures.

Local dermatitis may occur around the stoma in cats with prominent inguinal skin folds. Cats should be monitored long-term for urinary tract infection.

Based on a procedure of Mendham JH: A description and evaluation of antepubic urethrostomy in the male cat. J Small Anim Pract 11:709, 1970.

Plate 86
Approach to the Prepubic Urethra: Feline

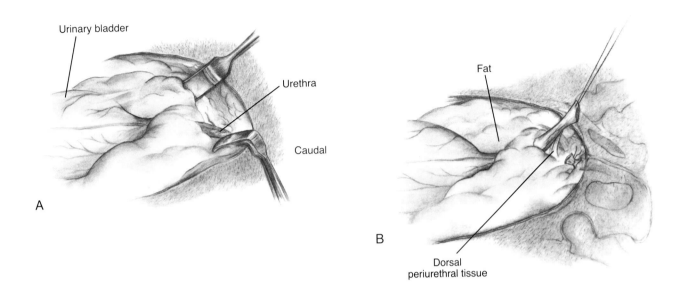

A

Urinary bladder

Urethra

Caudal

Fat

Dorsal
periurethral tissue

B

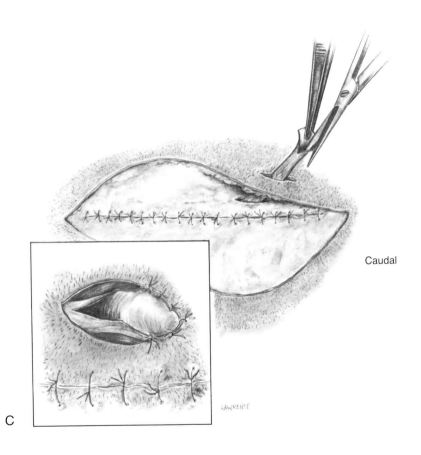

Caudal

C

Approach to the Testicles: Feline

INDICATIONS

Elective castration and as a component of perineal urethrostomy surgery.

DESCRIPTION OF THE PROCEDURE

A. The patient is positioned in lateral or dorsal recumbency, and the scrotal hair is plucked or shaved. A separate skin incision is made in a dorsal-ventral direction over each testicle to expose the visceral vaginal tunic. The testicle is exposed by digital pressure.

B. Excess subcutaneous fat and fascia are manually stripped from the spermatic cord. The spermatic cord is ligated with absorbable suture, and the testicle is excised distal to the ligature to complete the closed castration. Alternatively, an open castration begins with incision and stripping of the parietal vaginal tunic from the testicle and the spermatic cord. The ductus deferens is transected with scissors near the testicle. The ductus deferens and spermatic vessels are tied to provide hemostasis (inset), and the spermatic cord is transected distal to the ligation.

CLOSURE

The incisions in the scrotum are not sutured.

COMMENTS

A fenestrated rubber dam is used to exclude hair from the surgical field.

Many surgical techniques have been used successfully to neuter the cat. The authors do not recommend manual avulsion of the testicle and the spermatic cord.

Plate 87
Approach to the Testicles: Feline

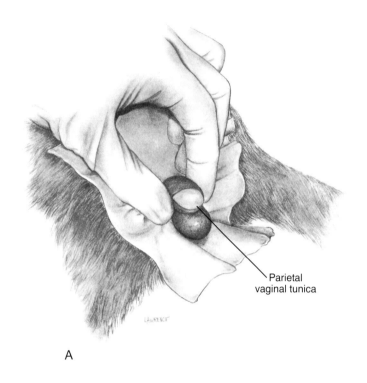

Parietal
vaginal tunica

A

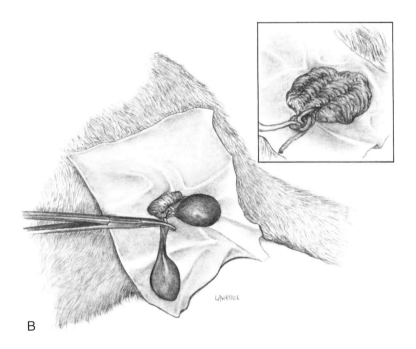

B

Approach to the Anal Sacs: Canine

INDICATIONS

Anal sacculectomy for chronic anal sacculitis, recurrent impaction, neoplasia, and ancillary surgical therapy for perianal fistulas.

DESCRIPTION OF THE PROCEDURE

A. The patient is positioned in ventral recumbency, with the rear limbs over the end of the operating table. The cranial thigh region is well padded to prevent pressure on the femoral nerve. The tail is directed cranially and maintained with tape. Open anal sacculectomy begins with insertion of the blade of dissecting scissors into the opening of the anal sac duct, located at the 4- and 8-o'clock positions of the anus. The blade is advanced to the full depth of the anal sac, and the anal sac and the duct are incised. The gray mucosal lining of the anal sac is exposed, and tissue forceps are applied for tissue traction to facilitate blunt and sharp dissection of the anal sac from the external anal sphincter muscle.

B. The closed technique is initiated with a vertical curved skin incision made directly over the anal sac. Subcutaneous tissues are separated, and the fibers of the external anal sphincter are visualized.

C. A combination of blunt and sharp dissection is used to carefully separate fibers of the external anal sphincter muscle, allowing identification of the anal sac. The surgeon dissects the anal sac from the surrounding muscle using blunt and sharp dissection, staying near the surface of the anal sac. Blood is supplied to the anal sac by a branch of the caudal rectal artery, located craniomedially. This branch is ligated or cauterized. The anal sac and the duct are dissected free, and the duct is ligated with absorbable suture close to its opening in the anus.

CLOSURE

The surgical site is lavaged with chlorhexidine or povidone-iodine solution. The subcutaneous tissues are apposed with absorbable suture in a continuous or interrupted pattern. The skin is closed with nonabsorbable suture in a simple interrupted pattern.

COMMENTS

The excised anal sacs are submitted for histopathologic examination.

When performing the closed technique, some surgeons prefer packing the anal sacs (e.g., with dental latex or melted paraffin) to facilitate identification of the sacs during dissection.

Complications of anal sacculectomy may include incisional dehiscence, chronic fistula formation, and fecal incontinence. Chronic fistula formation results from incomplete excision of the anal sac and its duct. Fecal incontinence is caused by excessive trauma to the external anal sphincter muscle or damage to the caudal rectal branch of the pudendal nerve. Meticulous surgical technique, including good hemostasis and gentle dissection close to the anal sac wall, will minimize complications.

Plate 88
Approach to the Anal Sacs: Canine

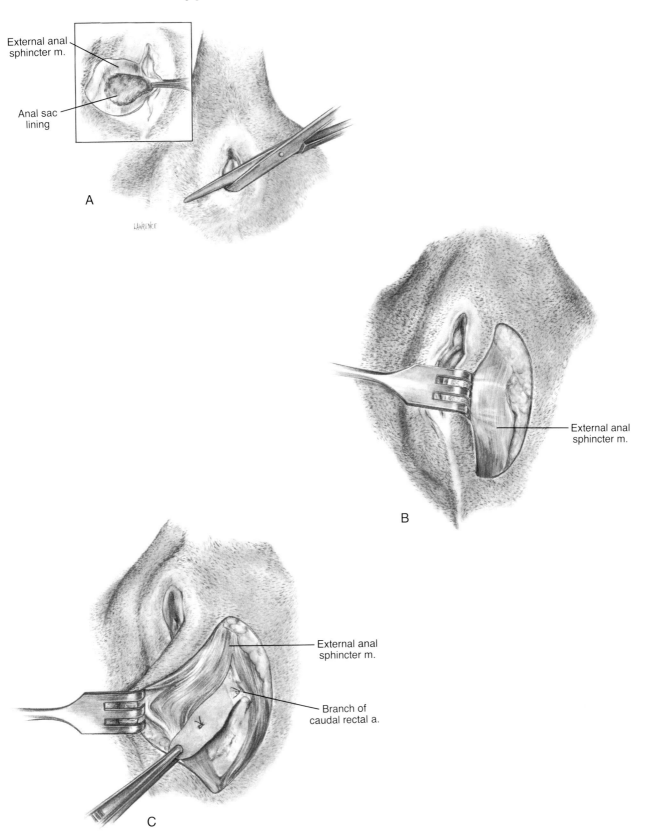

External anal
sphincter m.

Anal sac
lining

A

LAWRENCE

External anal
sphincter m.

B

External anal
sphincter m.

Branch of
caudal rectal a.

C

Muscular and Vascular Surgery

Approach to the Insertion of the Infraspinatus Muscle

INDICATIONS

Infraspinatus muscle tenectomy for treatment of infraspinatus muscle contracture.

DESCRIPTION OF THE PROCEDURE

A. The patient is positioned in lateral recumbency. A craniolateral curved skin incision is made from the midpoint of the scapular spine extending over the acromial process to the midshaft of the humerus.

B. The subcutaneous fat is incised, and the cephalic vein is ligated. The acromial head of the deltoid muscle is identified and subperiosteally elevated from the humeral shaft, facilitating its caudal retraction. This retraction exposes the tendons of insertion of the infraspinatus muscle proximally and the teres minor muscle distally. A combination of blunt and sharp dissection is used to free the tendon as it crosses the scapulohumeral joint. The tendon is excised, and the scapulohumeral joint is adducted to ensure increased range of motion.

CLOSURE

The subcutaneous tissue is closed with absorbable suture in a continuous pattern, and the skin is closed with nonabsorbable suture in an interrupted pattern.

COMMENTS

The affected leg is not immobilized; however, exercise is restricted for 2 weeks postoperatively.

This rare disorder has been described most commonly in hunting dogs, and the affected limb has a characteristic adducted elbow. The antebrachium is externally rotated and abducted. Increased range of motion of the shoulder should be evident following surgery.

Based on a procedure of Hufford T, Olmsted ML, and Butler HC: Contracture of the infraspinatus muscle and surgical correction in two dogs. J Am Anim Hosp Assoc 11:613, 1975.

Plate 89

Approach to the Insertion of the Infraspinatus Muscle

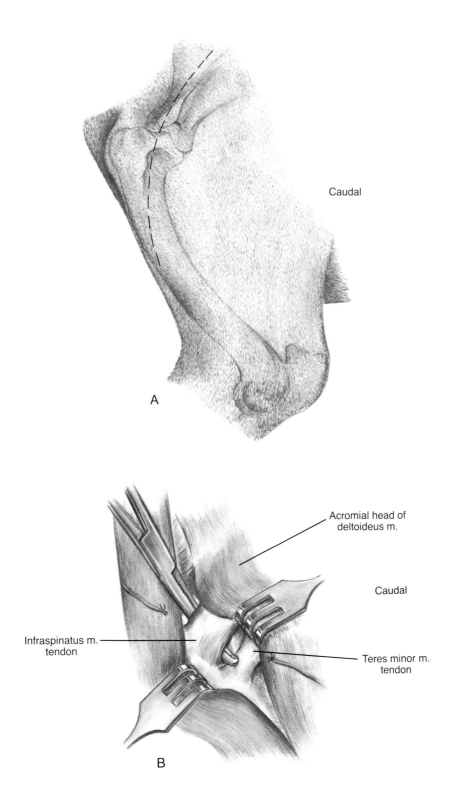

Approach to the Inguinal Ring

INDICATIONS

Inguinal herniorrhaphy in females and scrotal herniorrhaphy in males.

DESCRIPTION OF THE PROCEDURE

A. The patient is positioned in dorsal recumbency, and the four limbs are secured to the operating table. A caudoventral midline skin incision is made beginning at the umbilical scar cranially and extending to the level of the pecten ossis pubis caudally.

B. Subcutaneous tissues are sharply incised to expose the linea alba and external rectus abdominis muscle fascia. Mammary tissue is undermined by dissection on the external rectus abdominis muscle fascia and retracted laterally, exposing the inguinal ring.

Plate 90

Approach to the Inguinal Ring

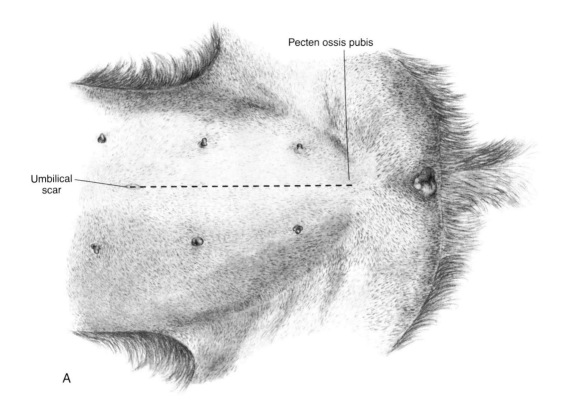

Pecten ossis pubis

Umbilical
scar

A

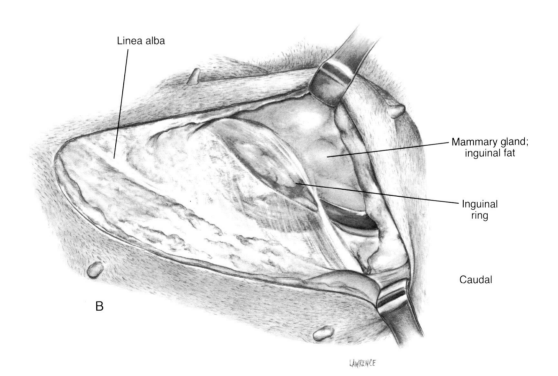

Linea alba

Mammary gland;
inguinal fat

Inguinal
ring

Caudal

B

LAWRENCE

Approach to the Inguinal Ring *continued*

DESCRIPTION OF THE PROCEDURE *continued*

C. The external inguinal ring is a slit in the aponeurosis of the external abdominal oblique muscle. When a hernia is present, the hernia sac is freed from subcutaneous tissue and opened to expose its contents. Abdominal viscera are returned to the abdominal cavity, and the hernia sac is excised at its base. In some cases, it is necessary to incise the inguinal ring cranially to allow hernia reduction. The external pudendal artery and vein and the genitofemoral nerve leave the ring caudomedially; compromise of these structures is avoided during ring closure. Nonabsorbable suture in a simple interrupted pattern is placed to appose the fasciae of the external abdominal oblique and external rectus abdominis muscles.

CLOSURE

Subcutaneous tissues are apposed with absorbable suture, after which the skin is closed with synthetic nonabsorbable suture in a simple interrupted pattern.

COMMENTS

Acquired inguinal hernias are most often seen in middle-aged females. Hernia contents may include the uterus, abdominal fat, the intestine, or the urinary bladder.

The contralateral inguinal ring should be examined intraoperatively so that small hernias that may not be palpable can be detected.

In performing herniorrhaphy in males, care is taken to not compromise the spermatic cord as it leaves the inguinal canal.

Plate 90

Approach to the Inguinal Ring *continued*

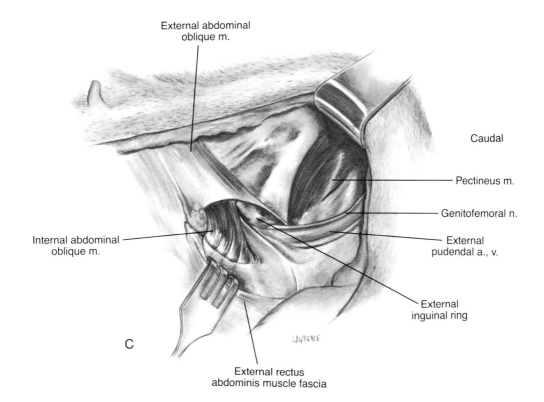

External abdominal oblique m.

Caudal

Pectineus m.

Genitofemoral n.

Internal abdominal oblique m.

External pudendal a., v.

External inguinal ring

C

LAWRENCE

External rectus abdominis muscle fascia

Approach to the Lateral Perineum

INDICATIONS

Perineal herniorrhaphy.

DESCRIPTION OF THE PROCEDURE

A. The patient is positioned in ventral recumbency, with the rear limbs over the end of the operating table. The cranial thigh region is well padded to prevent pressure on the femoral nerve. The tail is directed cranially, and a purse-string suture is placed in the anus. A curvilinear skin incision is made beginning lateral to the tail base and continuing to just ventral to the ischium.

B. After incising the subcutaneous fat, the surgeon opens the hernial sac, avoiding damage to any abdominal organs that may be present. Hernial contents are returned to the pelvic-abdominal cavity through the defect between the external anal sphincter and levator ani muscles. Fat may be excised or reduced, and reduction of hernia contents is maintained with a clamped, moistened gauze sponge. The pudendal nerve and the internal pudendal artery and vein are identified as they course over the ventrolateral surface of the coccygeus muscle and the dorsal surface of the internal obturator muscle.

Plate 91

Approach to the Lateral Perineum

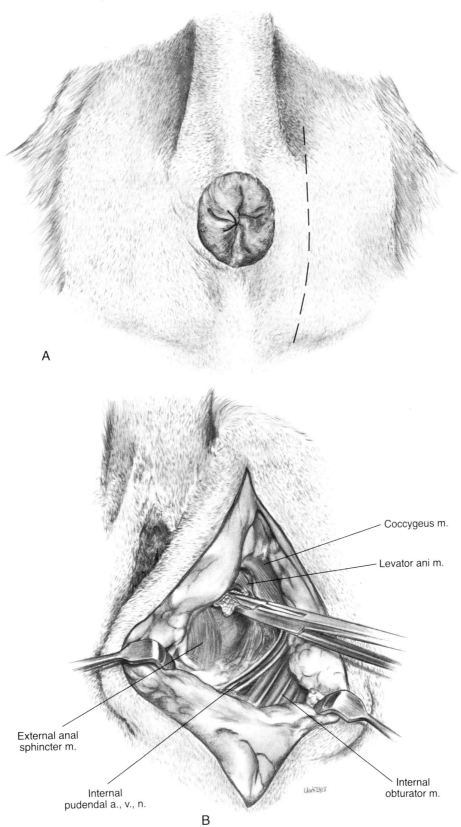

A

Coccygeus m.

Levator ani m.

External anal
sphincter m.

Internal
pudendal a., v., n.

Internal
obturator m.

LAWRENCE

B

Approach to the Lateral Perineum *continued*

DESCRIPTION OF THE PROCEDURE *continued*

C. The caudal and lateral borders of the internal obturator muscle and tendon are sharply incised at their origin on the ischium. A periosteal elevator is used to elevate the muscle belly from the ischium. Nonabsorbable suture in a simple interrupted pattern is placed between the external anal sphincter muscle and the internal obturator muscle caudally and between the coccygeus muscle and the internal obturator muscle cranially.

CLOSURE

The subcutaneous tissue is closed with absorbable suture in a continuous pattern, and the skin is closed with nonabsorbable suture in an interrupted pattern. The purse-string suture is removed from the anus, and a digital rectal examination is performed to ensure that sutures have not penetrated the rectum.

COMMENTS

A traditional method of perineal herniorrhaphy involves suturing the external anal sphincter, the coccygeus muscle, and the internal obturator muscle without obturator muscle elevation. The sacrotuberous ligament located craniolateral to the perineum has also been included in hernia reconstruction when the coccygeus muscle is atrophied. If the sacrotuberous ligament is used in herniorrhaphy, the surgeon should carefully place the suture through (rather than around) the ligament, avoiding the sciatic nerve located cranial to the ligament.

Many complications have been reported with perineal herniorrhaphy; however, most problems are avoided by careful attention to anatomic detail.

Castration is performed in conjunction with herniorrhaphy.

Bilateral herniorrhaphy may occasionally result in excessive tension on the external anal sphincter muscle. Bilateral injury to the pudendal nerve may result in fecal incontinence.

Based on procedures of Petit GD: Perineal hernia in the dog. Cornell Vet 52:261, 1962; and Earley TD, and Kolata RJ: Perineal hernia in the dog: an alternative method of correction. In Bojrab MJ (ed): Current Techniques in Small Animal Surgery. Philadelphia, Lea & Febiger, 1983, p 405.

Plate 91

Approach to the Lateral Perineum *continued*

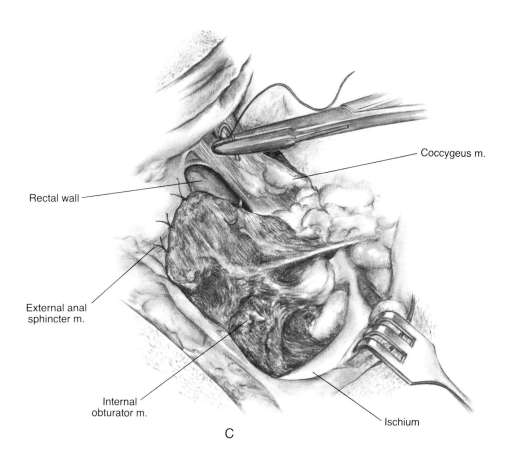

Coccygeus m.

Rectal wall

External anal
sphincter m.

Internal
obturator m.

Ischium

C

Approach to the Insertion of the Semitendinosus Muscle

INDICATIONS

Tenectomy for contracture of the semitendinosus muscle.

DESCRIPTION OF THE PROCEDURE

A. The patient is positioned in lateral recumbency, with the affected limb positioned toward the operating table. The medial aspect of the proximal crus is approached by a skin incision beginning from the caudal aspect of the medial femoral condyle proximally, continuing along the caudal aspect of the proximal tibia.

B. The gracilis and sartorius muscles are retracted following fascial incision. The contracted semitendinosus muscle insertion is visualized as it courses over the gastrocnemius muscle and inserts on the caudomedial aspect of the proximal tibia. Tenectomy of the area of insertion is performed.

CLOSURE

Fascia of the gracilis and sartorius muscles are apposed with synthetic absorbable suture in a simple interrupted pattern. The same suture and pattern are used to appose the subcutaneous tissues. The skin is closed with synthetic nonabsorbable suture in a simple interrupted pattern.

COMMENTS

This condition is similar to equine string-halt and has been diagnosed in German Shepherd dogs. The prognosis is guarded, since healing of the tenectomy usually results in recurrence of the contracture.

A similar surgical approach may be used for other muscles that may be affected, including the gracilis and semimembranosus muscles.

Plate 92

Approach to the Insertion of the Semitendinosus Muscle

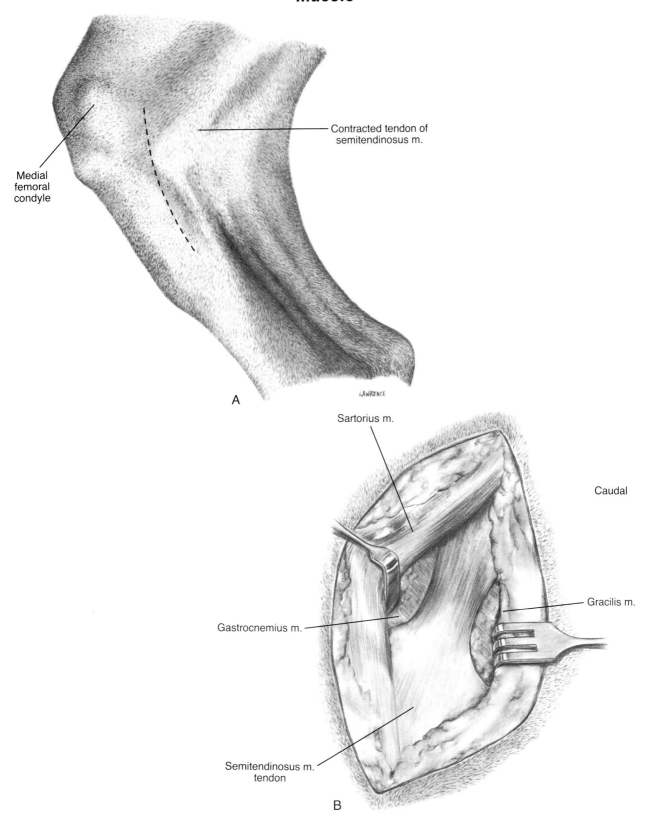

Medial femoral condyle

Contracted tendon of semitendinosus m.

LAWRENCE

A

Sartorius m.

Caudal

Gastrocnemius m.

Gracilis m.

Semitendinosus m. tendon

B

Approach to the Deep Digital Flexor Tendon: Feline

INDICATIONS

Deep digital flexor tenectomy as an alternative to onychectomy.

DESCRIPTION OF THE PROCEDURE

A. The patient is positioned in dorsal recumbency, and hair is clipped from the palmar surface of each paw. The paws are prepared for aseptic surgery, and a tourniquet is applied proximal to the elbow. A 5-mm skin incision is made beginning 3 to 5 mm proximal to the digital pad. The palmar digital vein is seen crossing the glistening, white surface of the tendon.

B. The tendon is bluntly isolated and elevated from the incision. A 5-mm section of the tendon is excised with a scalpel or scissors.

The procedure is performed on all five digits.

CLOSURE

The skin incision is closed with an absorbable suture in a simple interrupted pattern.

COMMENTS

The tourniquet is removed after application of a snug bandage from the paw to the distal antebrachium. Bandages are removed in 12 to 24 hours.

Shredded paper is used in place of litter to minimize wound contamination.

The technique described limits the cat's ability to scratch and is intended for cats whose owners object to amputation (onychectomy) of the third phalanx. Periodic nail trims are necessary to limit nail growth.

In the original description of the procedure, cyanoacrylate was used to appose skin.

Based on a procedure of Rife JN: Deep digital flexor tendonectomy: An alternative to amputation onychectomy for declawing cats. J Am Anim Hosp Assoc 24:73–76, 1988.

Plate 93
Approach to the Deep Digital Flexor Tendon: Feline

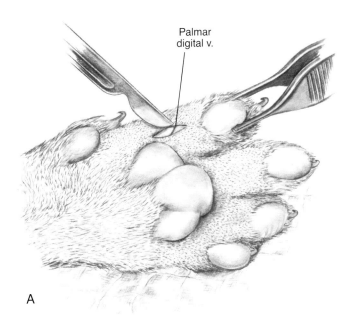

Palmar
digital v.

A

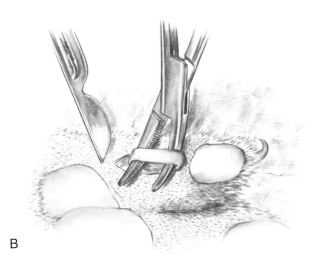

B

Approach to the Forequarter for Amputation

INDICATIONS

Amputation for neoplasia, congenital deformity, and neurologic or traumatic injuries causing permanent forelimb dysfunction.

DESCRIPTION OF THE PROCEDURE

A. The patient is positioned in lateral recumbency, with the affected limb positioned toward the surgeon. A teardrop-shaped skin incision is made beginning at the dorsal aspect of the scapula. At the acromial process of the scapula, the incision continues cranially and then medially through the axillary region, finally returning to the acromial process. Subcutaneous tissues are incised to expose the lateral superficial muscles of the shoulder.

Plate 94

Approach to the Forequarter for Amputation

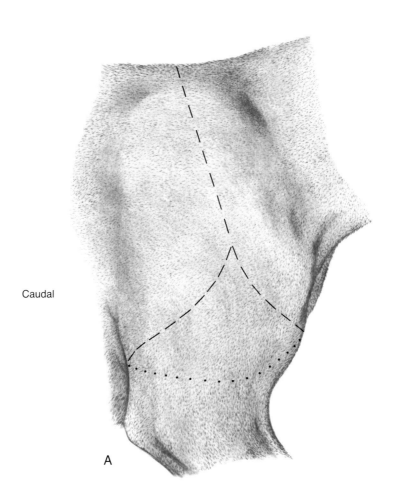

Caudal

A

Approach to the Forequarter for Amputation *continued*

DESCRIPTION OF THE PROCEDURE *continued*

B. The cervical portion of the trapezius and omotransversarius muscles are incised with dissection scissors at their attachment to the spine of the scapula.

Plate 94

Approach to the Forequarter for Amputation *continued*

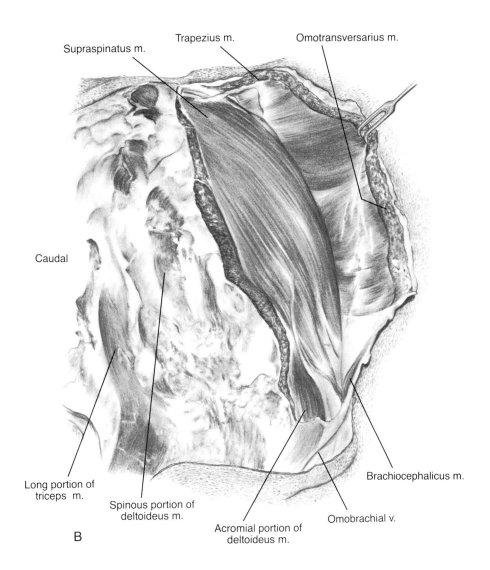

Supraspinatus m.

Trapezius m.

Omotransversarius m.

Caudal

Long portion of
triceps m.

Spinous portion of
deltoideus m.

Acromial portion of
deltoideus m.

Omobrachial v.

Brachiocephalicus m.

B

Approach to the Forequarter for Amputation *continued*

DESCRIPTION OF THE PROCEDURE *continued*

C. The cutaneus trunci and latissimus dorsi muscles are incised along the caudal aspect of the scapula. The thoracic portion of the trapezius muscle is elevated from the dorsal border of the scapula.

D. Placement of bone-holding forceps on the spine of the scapula allows lateral retraction, which aids elevation of the rhomboideus and serratus ventralis muscles from their attachment along the dorsal and medial aspects of the scapula.

Plate 94

Approach to the Forequarter for Amputation *continued*

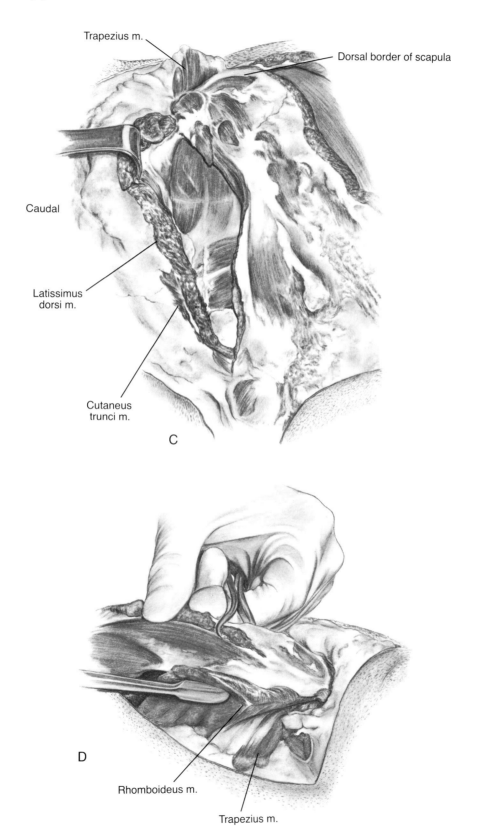

Trapezius m.

Dorsal border of scapula

Caudal

Latissimus
dorsi m.

Cutaneus
trunci m.

C

Rhomboideus m.

Trapezius m.

D

Approach to the Forequarter for Amputation *continued*

DESCRIPTION OF THE PROCEDURE *continued*

E. The forelimb is internally rotated, and the scapula is retracted laterally to expose the caudomedial aspect of the axillary space. Nerve roots of the brachial plexus are transected with dissection scissors. The axillary artery and vein are double-ligated and transected. The axillary lymph node is removed and submitted for biopsy if indicated. The deep pectoralis muscle is incised near its insertion on the humerus.

F. The forelimb is externally rotated to expose the craniolateral aspect of the shoulder. The omobrachial vein and the deltoid branch of the superficial cervical artery and vein are ligated and divided. The superficial pectoralis and brachiocephalicus muscles are incised near their insertion on the humerus. The cephalic vein, which lies beneath the brachiocephalicus muscle, is ligated and divided to complete the amputation.

CLOSURE

Wound closure begins by suturing fascia of the deep pectoral muscle to the scalenus muscle with absorbable suture in a simple interrupted pattern. Similar suture and pattern are used to appose fascia of the superficial pectoral and brachiocephalicus muscles; the deep pectoral fascia and the ventral latissimus dorsi muscle; the omotransversarius and trapezius muscles; and the dorsal latissimus dorsi. Sutures may be placed (tacked) in previously sutured muscle layers, and inverting interrupted Lembert sutures may be used to minimize dead space. Excess skin may be excised prior to apposition of subcutaneous tissues with absorbable suture in a simple interrupted pattern. The skin is apposed in a Y shape with nonabsorbable suture in a simple interrupted pattern.

COMMENTS

Wound drainage is usually not required, provided the primary wound is not contaminated and muscle closure minimizes potential dead space. Edema involving the ventral aspect of the wound is common.

A dog-ear appearance (excess skin at the wound corners) is a common postoperative result and should be corrected with plastic and reconstructive surgical techniques.

Postoperative bandage application is usually not required but may stabilize the wound and help decrease postoperative pain.

The authors recommend forequarter amputation rather than scapulohumeral disarticulation because of the cosmetically undesirable prominent scapula following muscle atrophy. Cosmesis is of less concern in long-haired dogs.

Scapulohumeral disarticulation is performed quickly and is recommended for debilitated patients unable to tolerate prolonged anesthesia, which may be required for forequarter amputation.

Based on a procedure of Harvey CE: Forequarter amputation in the dog and cat. J Am Anim Hosp Assoc 10:25, 1974.

Plate 94

Approach to the Forequarter for Amputation *continued*

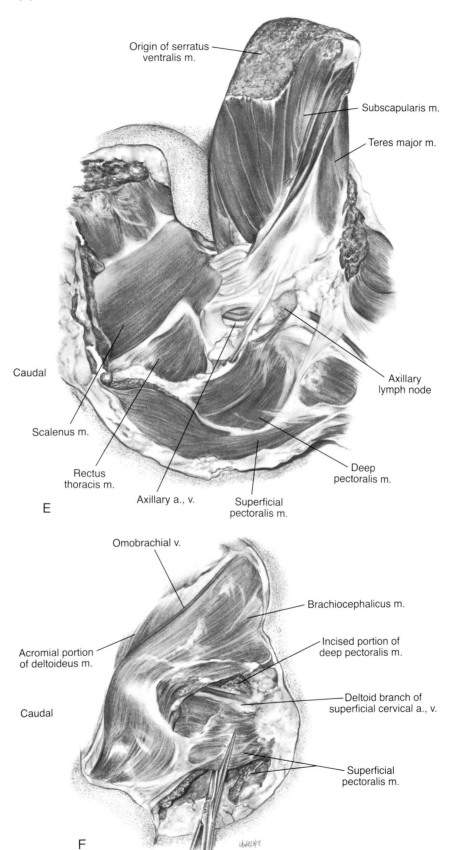

Origin of serratus ventralis m.

Subscapularis m.

Teres major m.

Caudal

Axillary lymph node

Scalenus m.

Rectus thoracis m.

Deep pectoralis m.

Axillary a., v.

Superficial pectoralis m.

E

Omobrachial v.

Brachiocephalicus m.

Acromial portion of deltoideus m.

Incised portion of deep pectoralis m.

Caudal

Deltoid branch of superficial cervical a., v.

Superficial pectoralis m.

F

LAWRENCE

317

Approach to the Forelimb for Amputation

INDICATIONS

Amputation for neoplasia, congenital deformity, and neurologic or traumatic injuries causing permanent forelimb dysfunction.

DESCRIPTION OF THE PROCEDURE

A. The patient is positioned in lateral recumbency, with the affected limb positioned toward the surgeon. A circumferential skin incision is made at the midbrachium between the olecranon and the acromion.

B. The subcutaneous tissues are incised to expose the superficial muscles of the proximal brachium. The omobrachial vein coursing lateral to the acromial portion of the deltoid muscle is divided and ligated or cauterized.

Approach to the Forelimb for Amputation

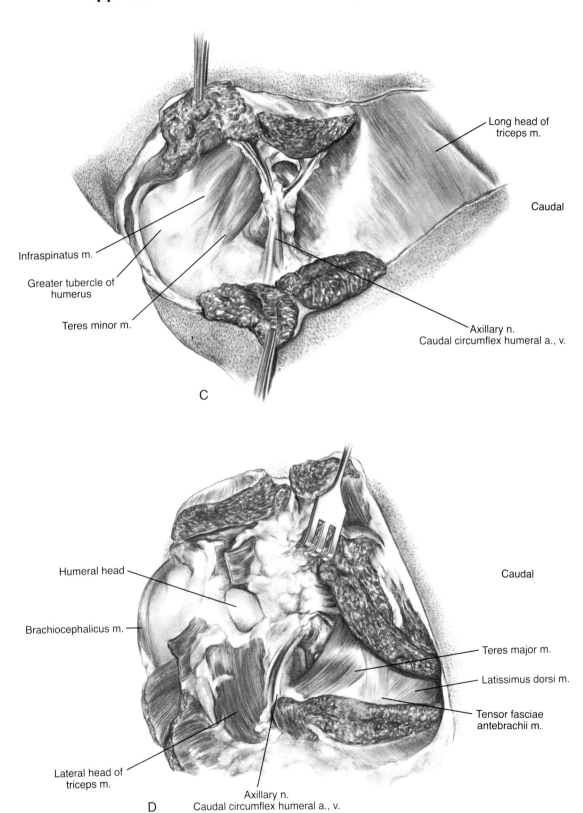

Long head of triceps m.

Caudal

Infraspinatus m.

Greater tubercle of humerus

Teres minor m.

Axillary n.
Caudal circumflex humeral a., v.

C

Humeral head

Caudal

Brachiocephalicus m.

Teres major m.

Latissimus dorsi m.

Tensor fasciae antebrachii m.

Lateral head of triceps m.

Axillary n.
Caudal circumflex humeral a., v.

D

Approach to the Forelimb for Amputation *continued*

DESCRIPTION OF THE PROCEDURE *continued*

E. The teres major and latissimus dorsi muscles are incised near their common insertion on the caudal aspect of the proximal humerus to expose neurovascular structures of the brachium. The brachial artery and vein are divided and ligated. The median, ulnar, and radial nerves are incised. The superficial and deep pectoralis muscles are incised near their insertion on the humerus. The musculocutaneous nerve and the coracobrachialis muscle are incised near the caudal aspect of the scapulohumeral joint.

F. Cranial and caudal scapulohumeral arthrotomy is performed, including incision of the tendinous insertions of the supraspinatus muscle cranially and the subscapularis muscle caudally. The brachium is internally rotated, exposing craniomedial structures of the scapulohumeral joint. The cephalic vein and the deltoid branch of the superficial cervical artery are divided and ligated. Amputation is completed by incision of the brachiocephalicus muscle, the medial joint capsule, and the biceps brachii muscle tendon of origin.

CLOSURE

Wound closure begins with suturing of the fascia of the latissimus dorsi muscle to the medial fascia of the long portion of the triceps muscle with absorbable suture in a simple interrupted pattern. Similar suture and pattern are used to appose the fascia of the superficial pectoralis muscle and the lateral fascia of the long portion of the triceps muscle. The brachiocephalicus muscle fascia is sutured along the cranial margin of the joined superficial pectoralis muscle and the long head of the triceps muscle. Sutures may be placed (tacked) in previously sutured muscle layers, and interrupted Lembert sutures may be used to minimize dead space. Excess skin may be excised prior to apposition of subcutaneous tissues with absorbable suture in a simple interupted pattern. The skin is apposed with nonabsorbable suture in a simple interrupted pattern.

COMMENTS

Wound drainage is usually not required, provided that the primary wound is not contaminated and muscle closure minimizes potential dead space. Edema involving the ventral aspect of the wound is common.

A dog-ear appearance (excess skin at the wound corners) is a common postoperative result and should be corrected with plastic and reconstructive surgical techniques.

Postoperative bandage application is not required but may stabilize the wound and help decrease postoperative pain.

The authors recommend forequarter amputation rather than scapulohumeral disarticulation because the cosmetically undesirable prominent scapula following muscle atrophy that is associated with the latter procedure does not occur with the former one. Cosmesis is of less concern in long-haired dogs.

Scapulohumeral disarticulation is performed quickly and is recommended for debilitated patients unable to tolerate prolonged anesthesia, which may be required for forequarter amputation.

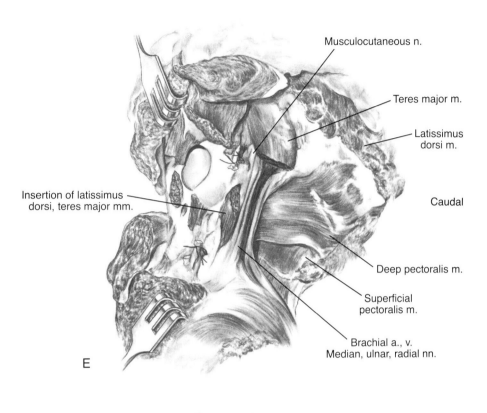

Musculocutaneous n.

Teres major m.

Latissimus dorsi m.

Insertion of latissimus dorsi, teres major mm.

Caudal

Deep pectoralis m.

Superficial pectoralis m.

Brachial a., v.
Median, ulnar, radial nn.

E

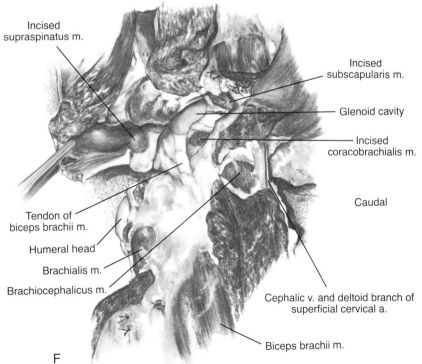

Incised supraspinatus m.

Incised subscapularis m.

Glenoid cavity

Incised coracobrachialis m.

Caudal

Tendon of biceps brachii m.

Humeral head

Brachialis m.

Brachiocephalicus m.

Cephalic v. and deltoid branch of superficial cervical a.

Biceps brachii m.

F

Approach to the Hindlimb for Amputation

INDICATIONS

Amputation for neoplasia, congenital deformity, and neourologic or traumatic injuries causing permanent hindlimb dysfunction.

DESCRIPTION OF THE PROCEDURE

A. The patient is positioned in lateral recumbency, with the affected limb positioned toward the surgeon. A circumferential skin incision is made at the distal third of the thigh, proximal to the patella.

B. The biceps femoris, tensor fasciae latae, sartorius, and quadriceps (vastus lateralis, medialis, intermedius, and rectus femoris) muscles are incised with dissection scissors or electrosurgical instruments.

C. The sciatic nerve is transected and retracted with the biceps femoris muscle. The femoral artery and vein are double-ligated at a location between the adductor and semimembranosus muscles. Myotomies of the adductor, semimembranosus, semitendinosus, caudal crural abductor, and gracilis muscles precede proximal-third femoral osteotomy. Osteotomy is performed with an osteotome and a mallet, an oscillating bone saw, or a wire saw. The amputation is completed by incision of the remaining portion of the caudal sartorius, pectineus fascia, and medial subcutaneous tissues.

Plate 90

Approach to the Hindlimb for Amputation

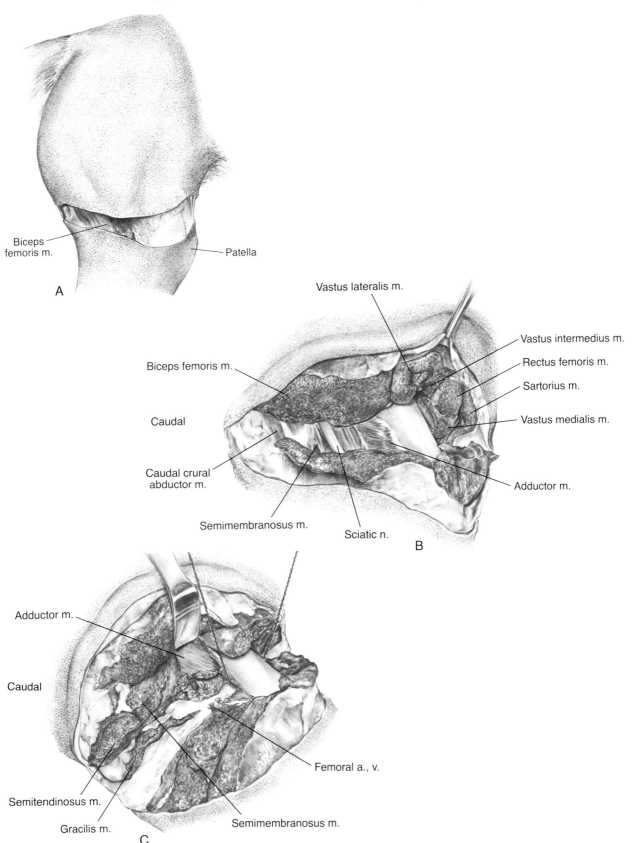

A

Biceps femoris m.

Patella

B

Vastus lateralis m.

Vastus intermedius m.

Rectus femoris m.

Sartorius m.

Vastus medialis m.

Biceps femoris m.

Caudal

Adductor m.

Caudal crural abductor m.

Semimembranosus m.

Sciatic n.

C

Adductor m.

Caudal

Femoral a., v.

Semitendinosus m.

Gracilis m.

Semimembranosus m.

Approach to the Hindlimb for Amputation *continued*

DESCRIPTION OF THE PROCEDURE *continued*

D. Amputation including coxofemoral disarticulation may be performed according to the previously described approach. Following muscle dissection performed as illustrated in Figure *C,* a sharp periosteal elevator is used to elevate the adductor and quadricep muscles (except the rectus femoris muscle) from their attachments on the femur.

E. Dissection scissors are used to incise the superficial, middle, and deep gluteal muscles; the internal and external obturator muscles; and the gemelli muscles at their attachments on the proximal femur and greater trochanter. Coxofemoral disarticulation is performed by incision of the joint capsule and the ligament of the head of the femur.

CLOSURE

Wound closure is the same for both proximal-third femur amputation and coxofemoral disarticulation. Fascia of the quadriceps musculature is apposed to the adductor muscle with synthetic absorbable suture in an interrupted Lembert pattern. For proximal-third femur amputation, this aspect of wound closure aids hemostasis at the femoral osteotomy site. Wound closure is continued by apposition of the gracilis and caudal sartorius muscles to the biceps femoris muscle with similar suture and pattern. Excess skin may be excised, followed by closure of the subcutaneous tissues with synthetic absorbable suture in a simple interrupted pattern. The skin is apposed with nonabsorbable suture in a simple interrupted pattern.

COMMENTS

Location of femoral artery and vein ligation and collateral circulation allows distal myotomy and proximal femoral elevation of the vastus lateralis, medialis, and intermedius muscles.

Wound drainage is usually not required, provided the primary wound is not contaminated and the inverting suture pattern used minimizes potential dead space.

A dog-ear appearance (excess skin at the wound corners) is a common postoperative result and should be corrected with plastic and reconstructive surgical techniques.

Postoperative bandage application is usually not required and may be difficult to maintain and keep clean.

An extended muscular stump following amputation in male dogs may cover the lateral aspect of the scrotum and the prepuce and thus provide better cosmesis than coxofemoral disarticulation does.

The authors recommend coxofemoral disarticulation for primary neoplasms affecting the femur, since it is difficult to detect intramedullary spread of the neoplasm to more proximal regions of the femur.

Plate 96
Approach to the Hindlimb for Amputation *continued*

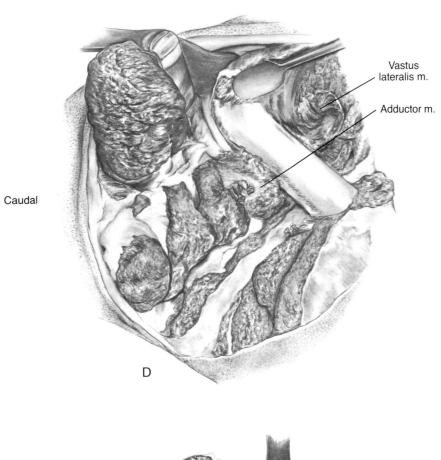

Vastus
lateralis m.

Adductor m.

Caudal

D

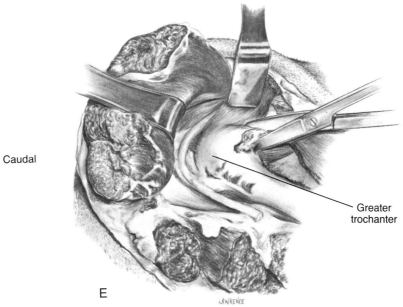

Caudal

Greater
trochanter

E

Approach to the Tail for Amputation

INDICATIONS

Amputation for neoplasia, congenital deformity, or traumatic injury causing permanent vascular compromise or dysfunction.

DESCRIPTION OF THE PROCEDURE

A. A purse-string suture is placed in the anus, and the patient is positioned in ventral recumbency. The skin of the tail is drawn forward toward the body, and incisions are made to form dorsal and ventral skin flaps.

B. Caudal vertebral disarticulation is performed with large dissection scissors or a scalpel blade concurrently with myotomy of tail musculature. Alternatively, vertebral osteotomy may be performed with bone cutters following myotomy. The two dorsal lateral caudal arteries and the median caudal artery usually require ligation. Direct pressure usually provides venous hemostasis.

CLOSURE

The subcutaneous tissues are apposed with synthetic absorbable suture in a simple interrupted pattern. The skin is apposed with nonabsorbable suture in a simple interrupted pattern.

COMMENTS

A compressive bandage may be difficult to maintain and is usually not necessary.

The authors prefer bone cutters for amputation because use of this instrument, unlike incision with a sharp scalpel and disarticulation, provides favorable hemostasis. Negative clinical results have not been reported for vertebral body osteotomy versus disarticulation.

Painful neuroma following tail amputation is rarely diagnosed.

Plate 97
Approach to the Tail for Amputation

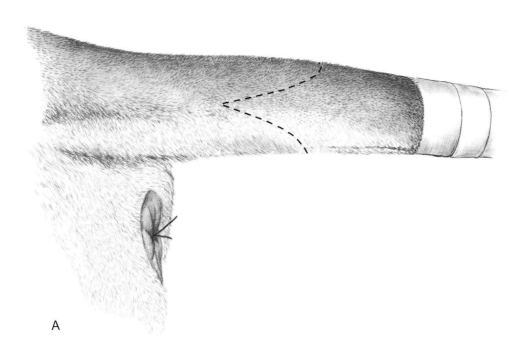

A

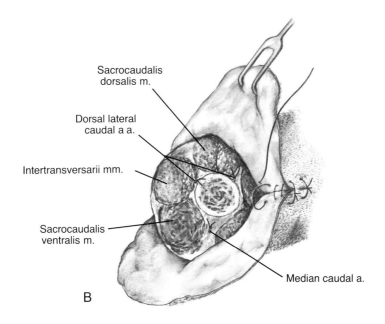

Sacrocaudalis
dorsalis m.

Dorsal lateral
caudal a a.

Intertransversarii mm.

Sacrocaudalis
ventralis m.

Median caudal a.

B

Approach to the Dewclaw for Amputation

INDICATIONS

Amputation for cosmesis, or to avoid injury to the dewclaw in hunting or performance dogs.

DESCRIPTION OF THE PROCEDURE

A. The patient is positioned in lateral recumbency. A narrow elliptical incision is made around the base of the dewclaw and over the proximal phalanx. The incision is made close to the dewclaw along the lateral aspect to ensure adequate skin for closure without tension.

B. A bone-holding forceps is placed on the unguis to aid medial retraction of the proximal and distal phalanges. Subcutaneous tissues are incised and a scalpel blade is used to disarticulate the metacarpophalangeal joint. Remaining tissues are incised, and hemorrhage from the dorsal common digital and palmar proper digital arteries is controlled by ligation or electrocoagulation.

CLOSURE

Subcutaneous tissues are apposed using synthetic absorbable suture in a simple interrupted pattern. The skin is apposed with nonabsorbable suture in a simple interrupted pattern.

COMMENTS

A bandage to prevent self-trauma is maintained until the skin sutures are removed.

A beveled osteotomy at the midbody of the first metacarpal may be performed as a component of the amputation to provide a smooth bony transition along the medial metacarpal area.

Large dissecting scissors may be used for the skin incision and disarticulation.

Dewclaws of the hindfeet are removed similarly; however, because bony development is incomplete, only soft tissue dissection is required.

Plate 98

Approach to the Dewclaw for Amputation

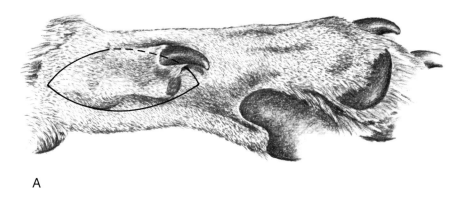

A

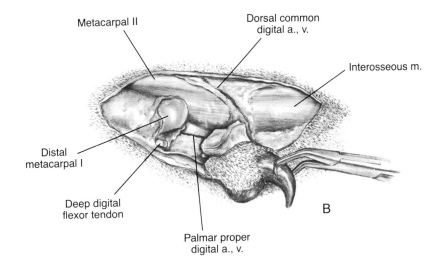

Metacarpal II

Dorsal common
digital a., v.

Interosseous m.

Distal
metacarpal I

Deep digital
flexor tendon

Palmar proper
digital a., v.

B

Approach to the Third Phalanx for Amputation: Feline

INDICATIONS

Elective onychectomy and trauma or infection involving the third phalanx.

DESCRIPTION OF THE PROCEDURE

A. The patient is positioned in lateral recumbency, and a tourniquet is applied proximal to the elbow. The entire paw is prepared with surgical scrub; however, hair clipping is not necessary. The nail is extended with tissue forceps or by dorsal pressure on the footpad. A no. 11 scalpel blade is used to completely excise the third phalanx by severing all its ligament and tendon attachments. Complete excision is achieved by careful dissection, including the dorsal and ventral ungual crest (inset). The digital pad should not be injured, and the articular surface of the second phalanx should be clearly visible (see Fig. *B,* inset) following excision of the phalanx.

B. Alternatively, a nail trimmer is positioned between the ungual crest and the second phalanx, with care being taken to exclude the digital footpad. Following excision of the phalanx, the wound should be examined and the articular surface of the second phalanx should be visible. A small palmar portion of the ventral ungual crest (inset) may remain following excision with nail trimmers.

CLOSURE

Skin closure with absorbable suture is optional. The authors do not recommend use of cyanoacrylates for wound closure.

COMMENTS

The tourniquet is removed after application of a snug bandage from the paw to the midantebrachium. Excessive tension (tightening) of the bandage may compromise vascular supply to the extremity. Bandages are removed in 12 to 24 hours.

Shredded paper is used in place of litter to minimize wound contamination.

If the dorsal ungual crest is not excised, partial claw regrowth may occur, requiring reoperation.

Plate 99

Approach to the Third Phalanx for Amputation: Feline

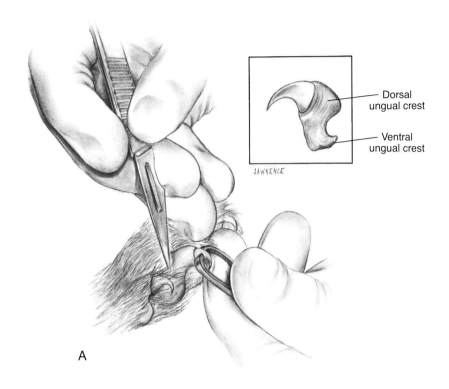

Dorsal ungual crest

Ventral ungual crest

A

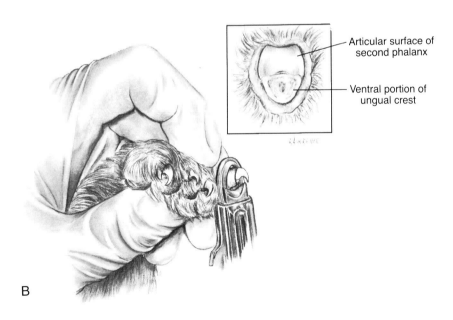

Articular surface of second phalanx

Ventral portion of ungual crest

B

Approach to the Femoral Artery

INDICATIONS

Open approach for direct cardiac catheterization or hindlimb angiography.

DESCRIPTION OF THE PROCEDURE

A. The patient is positioned in dorsal or lateral recumbency, and the medial aspect of the proximal hindlimb is prepared for surgery. A skin incision is made on the cranial aspect of the body of the pectineus muscle.

B. The subcutaneous tissue is incised, and the femoral artery and vein are exposed just cranial to the body of the pectineus muscle. The femoral artery is located cranial to the vein. The vessels may be separated by blunt dissection prior to catheterization.

CLOSURE

The subcutaneous tissue is closed with absorbable suture in an interrupted or continuous pattern. The skin is closed with nonabsorbable suture in a simple interrupted pattern.

COMMENTS

Following angiography, the femoral artery is ligated prior to wound closure. The hindlimb is not compromised by vessel ligation.

Plate 100

Approach to the Femoral Artery

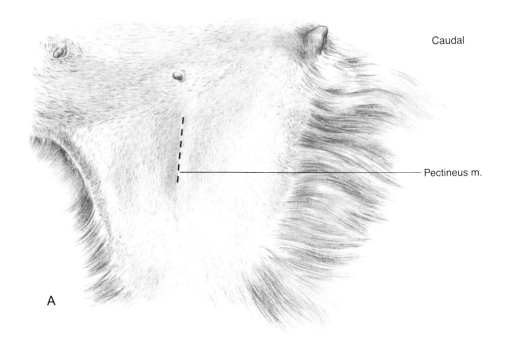

Caudal

Pectineus m.

A

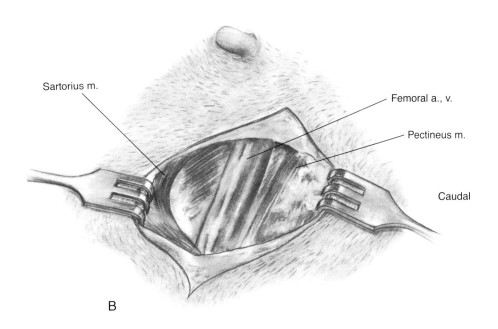

Sartorius m.

Femoral a., v.

Pectineus m.

Caudal

B

Approach to the Common Carotid Artery

INDICATIONS

Open approach for direct cardiac catheterization and cranial angiography.

DESCRIPTION OF THE PROCEDURE

A. The patient is positioned in right lateral recumbency. A skin incision is made over the external jugular vein caudal to the union of the maxillary and linguofacial veins.

B. The platysma muscle is incised parallel to the skin incision. The sternocephalicus muscle fibers are separated and retracted to expose the common carotid artery and the vagosympathetic trunk, bordered by the longus colli muscle dorsally and the sternothyroideus muscle ventrally. Cardiac catheterization from the left common carotid artery is performed by placement of a distal occlusive ligature and a proximal circumferential ligature around the artery and the catheter (inset).

CLOSURE

The common carotid artery is ligated following the procedure without adversely affecting the blood supply to distal areas. Silk suture is recommended for vessel ligation.

The skin incision is closed with synthetic nonabsorbable suture in a simple interrupted pattern. Sutures are spaced to allow catheter maintenance if required.

Plate 101

Approach to the Common Carotid Artery

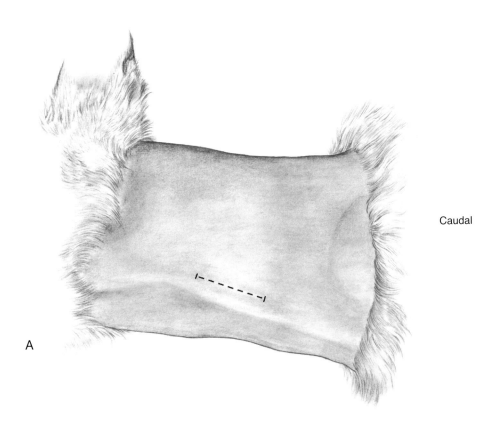

Caudal

A

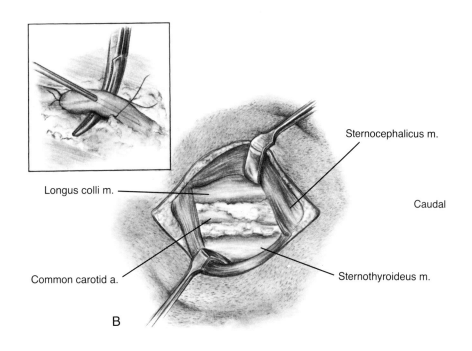

Sternocephalicus m.

Longus colli m.

Caudal

Common carotid a.

Sternothyroideus m.

B

Approach to the External Jugular Vein

INDICATIONS

Open approach for direct catheterization for fluid administration, parenteral alimentation, angiography, and venotomy for heartworm removal.

DESCRIPTION OF THE PROCEDURE

A. The patient is positioned in lateral recumbency. A skin incision is made over the external jugular vein caudal to the union of the maxillary and linguofacial veins.

B. The platysma muscle is incised parallel to the skin incision. The external jugular vein lies directly under the platysma muscle, paralleling the lateral aspect of the sternocephalicus muscle.

CLOSURE

The skin incision is closed with synthetic nonabsorbable suture in a simple interrupted pattern. Sutures are spaced to allow catheter maintenance if required.

COMMENTS

The external jugular vein is usually ligated following cardiac catheterization, since vessel ligation does not interfere with function.

External jugular venotomy for cardiac catheterization should be performed on the right side to avoid complications associated with persistent left cranial vena cava, a remote possibility.

Right external jugular venotomy for heartworm removal may be recommended in dogs with caval syndrome.

Plate 102
Approach to the External Jugular Vein

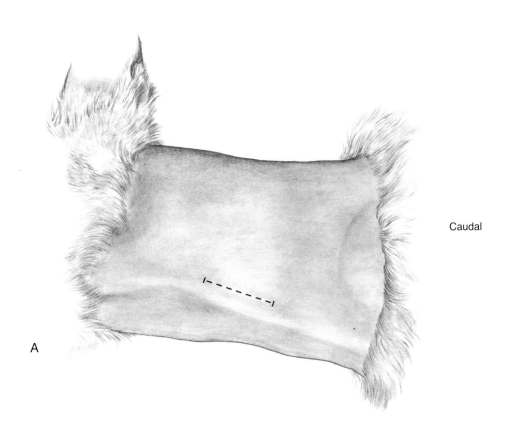

Caudal

A

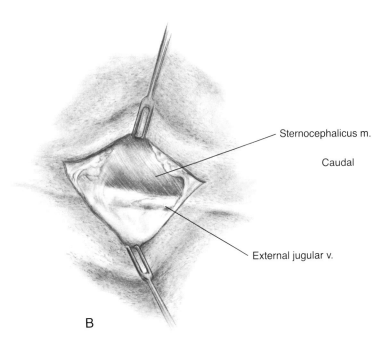

Sternocephalicus m.

Caudal

External jugular v.

B

Peripheral Nerve Surgery

Approach to the Brachial Plexus

INDICATIONS

Exploratory surgery for neoplasia affecting the brachial plexus.

DESCRIPTION OF THE PROCEDURE

A. The patient is positioned in lateral recumbency over a padded area (e.g., a rolled towel) to provide elevation of the operative area. A curved skin incision is made from the midpoint of the cranial border of the scapula to an area distal to the greater tubercle of the humerus.

B. Sharp dissection is performed with scissors to expose the strap-like omotransversarius and brachiocephalicus muscles. Omotransversarius myotomy is performed over the cranial border of the scapula.

Plate 103

Approach to the Brachial Plexus

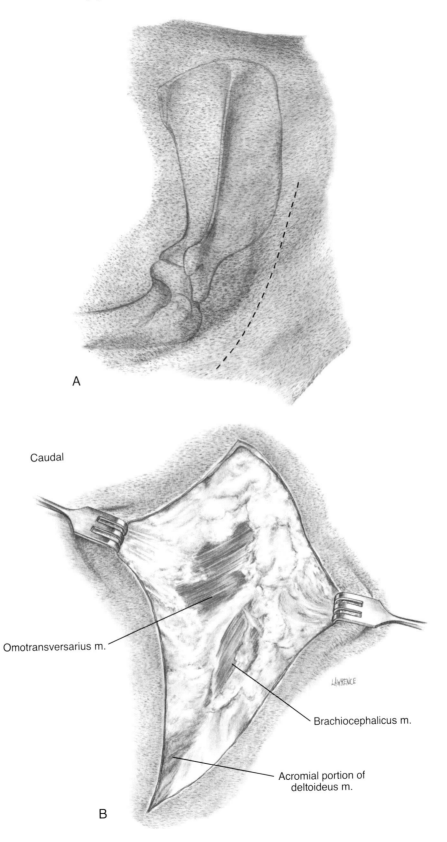

A

Caudal

Omotransversarius m.

Brachiocephalicus m.

Acromial portion of
deltoideus m.

B

Approach to the Brachial Plexus *continued*

DESCRIPTION OF THE PROCEDURE *continued*

C. Dissection is continued along the dorsolateral border of the brachiocephalicus muscle, which is retracted ventrally with the superficial cervical lymph node. The cranial border of the scapula and the omotransversarius muscle are retracted in a caudodorsal direction to provide craniodorsal exposure of the axilla. The supraspinous and ascending branches of the superficial cervical artery and vein are ligated and divided.

D. Subscapular fat and fascia are incised, exposing the axillary space. The superficial and deep portions of the scalenus muscle may be incised cranial to the first rib for exposure of components of the brachial plexus, including ventral branches of the seventh and eighth cervical and first thoracic nerves. The vessels and nerves of the thoracic inlet are avoided.

CLOSURE

A soft rubber drain is placed in the operative field and exited ventrally in the axilla to minimize potential dead space. The scalenus and omotransversarius muscles are apposed with synthetic absorbable suture in an interrupted cruciate mattress pattern. Subcutaneous tissues are apposed with synthetic absorbable suture in a simple interrupted pattern, then the skin is closed with nonabsorbable suture in a simple interrupted pattern.

COMMENTS

Fascicular nerve biopsy or resection of an affected portion of the brachial plexus may be performed after exploration of the axillary space.

Attempts to excise all of the neoplastic neural tissue are usually unsuccessful and invariably result in severe neurologic deficits. Neoplasms of the brachial plexus are locally invasive and are associated with a poor prognosis. Surgical exploration, radical resection of the neoplastic plexus, and forequarter amputation are recommended.

Based on a procedure of Sharp NJH: Craniolateral approach to the canine brachial plexus. Vet Surg 17:18, 1988.

Plate 103

Approach to the Brachial Plexus *continued*

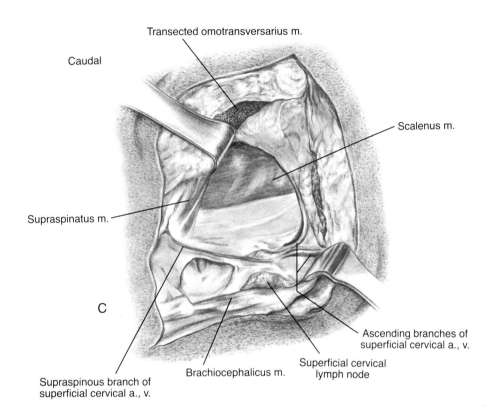

Caudal

Transected omotransversarius m.

Scalenus m.

Supraspinatus m.

C

Supraspinous branch of
superficial cervical a., v.

Brachiocephalicus m.

Superficial cervical
lymph node

Ascending branches of
superficial cervical a., v.

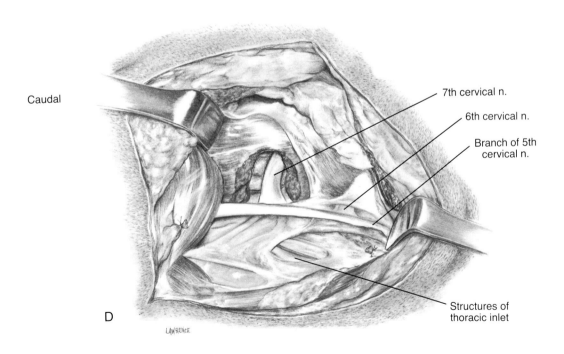

Caudal

7th cervical n.

6th cervical n.

Branch of 5th
cervical n.

Structures of
thoracic inlet

D

LAWRENCE

Approach to the Radial Nerve

INDICATIONS

Exploratory surgery for neurorrhaphy or nerve decompression related to fracture-associated trauma.

DESCRIPTION OF THE PROCEDURE

A. The patient is positioned in lateral recumbency. The skin is incised from the greater tubercle of the humerus proximally to the lateral epicondyle distally, following the craniolateral border of the humerus.

B. The subcutaneous fat and fascia are incised on the same line and retracted with skin. The fat and the brachial fascia are incised to allow visualization of the cephalic vein and the underlying musculature.

C. The proximal and distal aspects of the cephalic vein are ligated and divided. The brachial fascia is incised along the lateral border of the brachiocephalicus muscle, allowing retraction of the lateral head of the triceps muscle. The proximal radial nerve is medial to the lateral head of the triceps muscle and caudal to the brachialis muscle.

CLOSURE

Following radial nerve surgery, the superficial fascia of the brachialis muscle is apposed to the fascia of the brachiocephalicus and superficial pectoralis muscles with synthetic absorbable suture in a simple interrupted pattern. The same pattern and suture are used to appose the lateral head of the triceps muscle fascia to the deep brachial fascia and the subcutaneous tissues. The skin is closed with nonabsorbable suture in a simple interrupted pattern.

COMMENTS

The authors recommend review of neurorrhaphy techniques before exploratory surgery for radial nerve trauma.

Radial nerve dysfunction may be related to nerve compression from bony callus associated with acceptable fracture-healing or fibrous-like tissue associated with complicated healing (e.g., infection and nonunion). The proximal and distal aspects of the proximal radial nerve should be isolated and used to orient the surgeon toward the affected segment of nerve.

Based on a procedure of Piermattei DL, and Greeley RG: Approach to the shaft of the humerus. In Piermattei DL, and Greeley RG (eds): An Atlas of Surgical Approaches to the Bones of the Dog and Cat. Philadelphia, WB Saunders, 1979, p 82.

Plate 104
Approach to the Radial Nerve

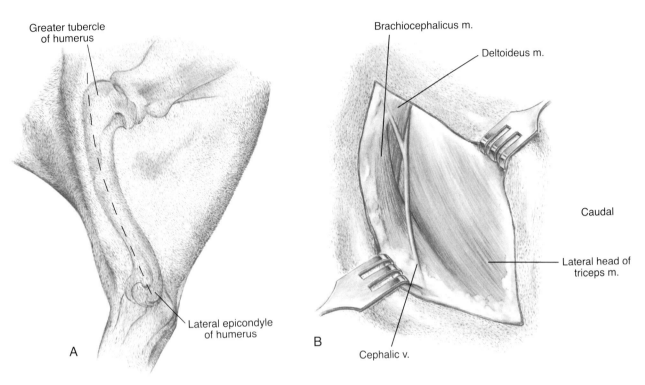

Greater tubercle
of humerus

Lateral epicondyle
of humerus

A

Brachiocephalicus m.

Deltoideus m.

Caudal

Lateral head of
triceps m.

B

Cephalic v.

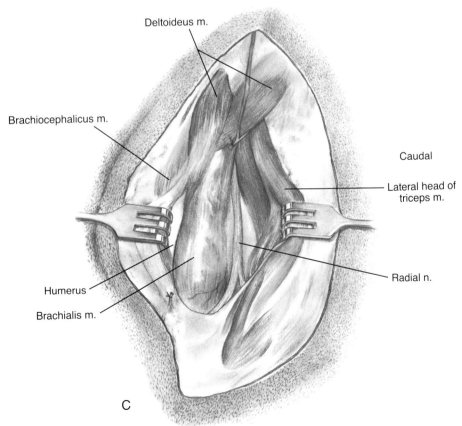

Deltoideus m.

Brachiocephalicus m.

Caudal

Lateral head of
triceps m.

Radial n.

Humerus

Brachialis m.

C

Approach to the Ulnar Nerve

INDICATIONS

Fascicular nerve biopsy as a diagnostic procedure for neuromuscular disease.

DESCRIPTION OF THE PROCEDURE

A. The patient is positioned in lateral recumbency. A 5-cm skin incision is centered on the medial epicondyle of the humerus.

B. The deep brachial fascia is incised on the cranial border of the medial head of the triceps muscle. The ulnar nerve crosses the elbow caudal to the medial epicondyle of the humerus. Retraction of the medial head of the triceps muscle allows visualization of the nerve as it courses between the superficial digital flexor and flexor carpi ulnaris muscles. Fascicular biopsy is performed by isolation of 30% to 50% of the nerve fascicles followed by transverse resection, while constant tension is provided on the fascicular biopsy specimen with suture or forceps.

CLOSURE

The deep brachial fascia and medial head of the triceps muscle fascia are apposed with synthetic, absorbable suture in a simple interrupted pattern. The same pattern and suture are used to appose the subcutaneous tissues. The skin is closed with nonabsorbable suture in a simple interrupted pattern.

COMMENTS

The authors recommend that the surgeon contact the receiving service laboratory to review techniques for fascicular biopsy specimen collection and handling.

Neurologic deficits related to fascicular biopsy are not expected.

Based on a procedure of Braund KG, Walker TL, and Vandevilde M: Fascicular nerve biopsy in the dog. Am J Vet Res 40:1025, 1979.

Plate 105
Approach to the Ulnar Nerve

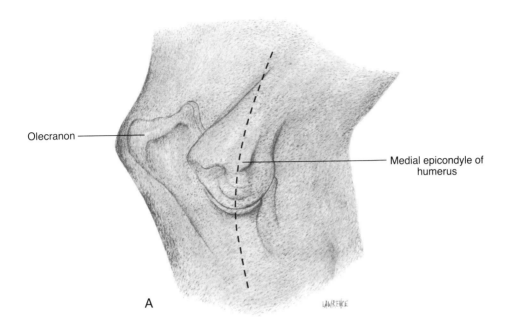

Olecranon

Medial epicondyle of
humerus

LAWRENCE

A

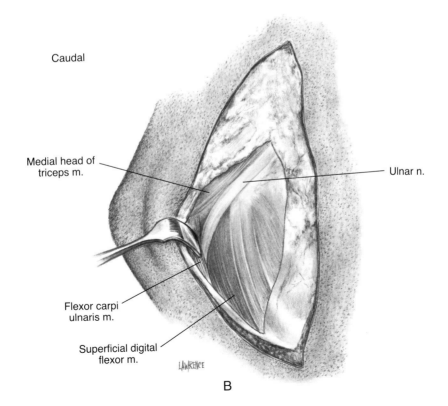

Caudal

Medial head of
triceps m.

Ulnar n.

Flexor carpi
ulnaris m.

Superficial digital
flexor m.

LAWRENCE

B

Approach to the Lumbosacral Nerve Trunk

INDICATIONS

Exploratory surgery for neurorrhaphy or nerve decompression related to fracture-associated trauma.

DESCRIPTION OF THE PROCEDURE

A. The patient is positioned in dorsal recumbency. A dorsal, paramidline skin incision is made from the craniodorsal iliac spine cranially to an area between the coxofemoral joint and the ischiatic tuberosity caudally.

B. The gluteal fascia is incised to expose the superficial gluteal and sacrospinalis muscles. The superficial gluteal muscle fascia is incised, and the sacrospinalis muscle fibers are separated directly over the palpable dorsal iliac spine and body.

C. Myotomy of the middle gluteal muscle is performed along the dorsal aspect of the ilial wing and body. Retraction of this muscle and the sacrospinalis muscle followed by blunt intrapelvic dissection exposes the lumbosacral nerve trunk. Cranial extension of the operative field allows observation of the cranial gluteal artery, vein, and nerve, which crosses the dorsal ilium just caudal to the sacroiliac joint.

CLOSURE

The middle and superficial gluteal muscle fascia are apposed with synthetic absorbable suture in a simple interrupted pattern. The same pattern and suture are used to appose the subcutaneous tissues. The skin is closed with nonabsorbable suture in a simple interrupted pattern.

COMMENTS

Lumbosacral nerve trunk injury may be related to bony callus associated with pelvic fracture healing. Surgery for lumbosacral nerve dysfunction may be combined with osteotomy procedures to improve pelvic canal diameter.

Plate 106

Approach to the Lumbosacral Nerve Trunk

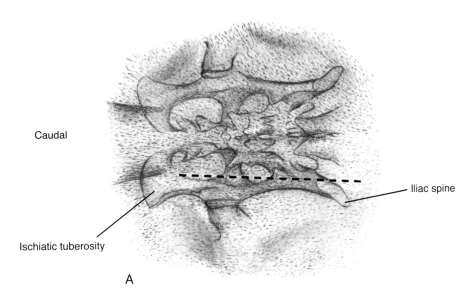

Caudal

Iliac spine

Ischiatic tuberosity

A

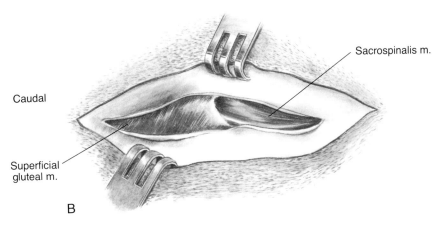

Caudal

Sacrospinalis m.

Superficial
gluteal m.

B

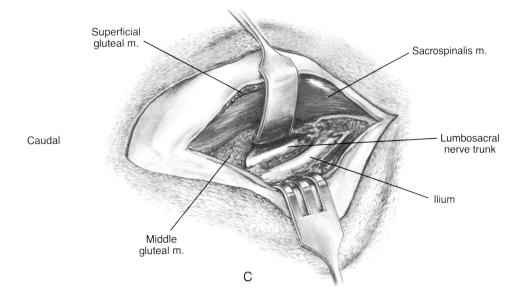

Superficial
gluteal m.

Sacrospinalis m.

Caudal

Lumbosacral
nerve trunk

Ilium

Middle
gluteal m.

C

Approach to the Sciatic Nerve

INDICATIONS

Exploratory surgery for neurorrhaphy or nerve decompression related to fracture-associated trauma; iatrogenic trauma as a complication of fracture repair, femoral head and neck ostectomy, or perineal herniorrhaphy.

DESCRIPTION OF THE PROCEDURE

A. The patient is positioned in lateral recumbency. A curvilinear skin incision is made caudal to the greater trochanter of the femur between this bony prominence and the ischiatic tuberosity.

B. The subcutaneous tissues are incised in line with the skin incision. The fascia of the biceps femoris muscle is incised along its cranial border with the tensor fasciae latae to allow visualization of the greater trochanter of the femur, the biceps femoris muscle, and the gluteal musculature.

C. Retraction of the superficial gluteal and biceps femoris muscles allows visualization of the sciatic nerve and the caudal gluteal artery and vein as they course over the gemelli and internal obturator muscles.

CLOSURE

The biceps femoris muscle fascia and the tensor fascia lata are apposed with synthetic absorbable suture in a simple interrupted pattern. The same pattern and suture are used to appose the subcutaneous tissues. The skin is closed with nonabsorbable suture in a simple interrupted pattern.

COMMENTS

Iatrogenic sciatic nerve entrapment associated with suture placement around the sacrotuberous ligament is a potential complication of perineal herniorrhaphy. Sciatic nerve exploration and decompression from a lateral approach is recommended to allow visualization of the entrapping suture and to avoid disruption of the perineal herniorrhaphy.

Plate 107

Approach to the Sciatic Nerve

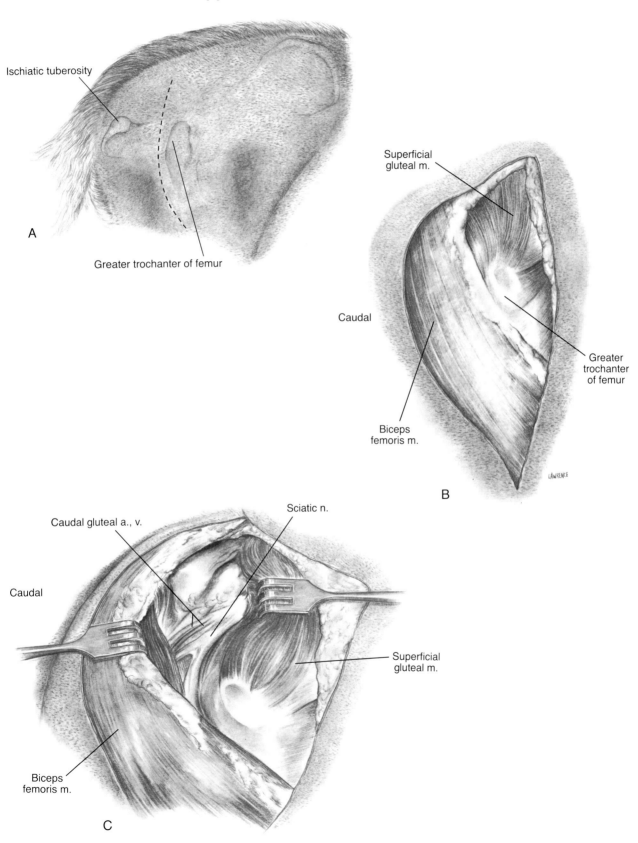

A

Ischiatic tuberosity

Greater trochanter of femur

B

Superficial gluteal m.

Caudal

Biceps femoris m.

Greater trochanter of femur

LAWRENCE

C

Caudal gluteal a., v.

Sciatic n.

Caudal

Superficial gluteal m.

Biceps femoris m.

Approach to the Peroneal Nerve

INDICATIONS

Fascicular nerve biopsy as a diagnostic procedure for neuromuscular disease.

DESCRIPTION OF THE PROCEDURE

A. The patient is positioned in lateral recumbency. A 5-cm skin incision is made from the lateral condyle of the femur to a point distal to the tibial tuberosity.

B. The biceps femoris muscle fascia is incised parallel to muscle fibers at the level between the patella and the tibial tuberosity. The fascia and the muscle fibers are divided to the level of the gastrocnemius muscle. The peroneal nerve courses over the lateral aspect of this muscle and divides into deep and superficial portions between the gastrocnemius and peroneus longus muscles. Fascicular biopsy is performed by isolation of 30% to 50% of the nerve fascicles followed by transverse resection, while constant tension is provided on the fascicular biopsy specimen with suture or forceps.

CLOSURE

The biceps femoris muscle fascia is apposed with synthetic absorbable suture in a simple interrupted pattern. The same pattern and suture are used to appose the subcutaneous tissues. The skin is closed with nonabsorbable suture in a simple interrupted pattern.

COMMENTS

The authors recommend that the surgeon contact the receiving service laboratory to review techniques for fascicular biopsy specimen collection and handling.

Neurologic deficits related to fascicular biopsy are not expected.

Based on a procedure of Braund KG, Walker TL, and Vandevelde M: Fascicular nerve biopsy in the dog. Am J Vet Res 40:1025, 1979.

Plate 108
Approach to the Peroneal Nerve

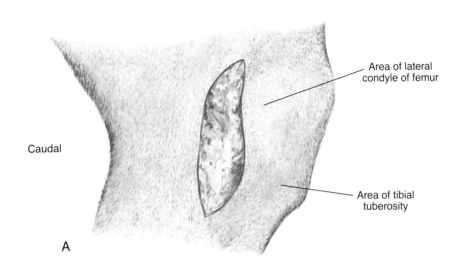

Area of lateral
condyle of femur

Caudal

Area of tibial
tuberosity

A

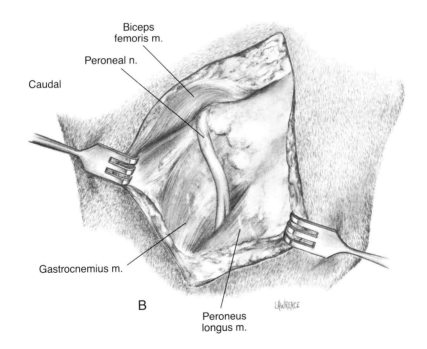

Biceps
femoris m.

Peroneal n.

Caudal

Gastrocnemius m.

B

Peroneus
longus m.

Plastic and Reconstructive Surgery

Approach to the Caudal Auricular Artery

INDICATIONS

Axial pattern flap for wound reconstruction involving the head and neck.

DESCRIPTION OF THE PROCEDURE

A. The patient is positioned in lateral recumbency, with the scapula positioned perpendicular to the long axis of the body. The skin flap base is centered over the lateral aspect of the wing of the atlas. The cranial border of the flap is marked by a palpable depression between the wing of the atlas and the vertical ear canal. Dorsal and ventral parallel skin incisions are made on the lateral aspect of the neck extending caudally to the scapula.

B. The surgeon joins the skin incisions and elevates the flap from caudal to cranial with dissecting scissors, staying deep to the subcutaneous tissues and platysma muscle. Care is taken to not disturb the branches of the caudal auricular artery and vein, which enter the flap at its cranial aspect.

CLOSURE

The donor site is closed by apposition of the subcutaneous tissue with absorbable suture in an interrupted or a continuous pattern. The skin is closed with nonabsorbable suture in a simple interrupted pattern. A soft rubber drain is placed in the wound, and the flap is sutured into the wound defect with nonabsorbable suture in a simple interrupted pattern. A subcutaneous closure is not performed on the flap to avoid possible compromise of vascular supply to the flap edges.

COMMENTS

A bridge incision is made between the donor bed and the wound site.

Owing to variations in the length and number of the vascular branches, necrosis may affect 10% to 30% of the length of the flap. The flap does not necessarily extend to the scapula; shorter flaps have greater viability.

Based on a procedure of Smith MM, Payne JT, Moon M, and Freeman LE: Axial pattern flap based on the caudal auricular artery in dogs. Am J Vet Res 52:992, 1991.

Plate 109
Approach to the Caudal Auricular Artery

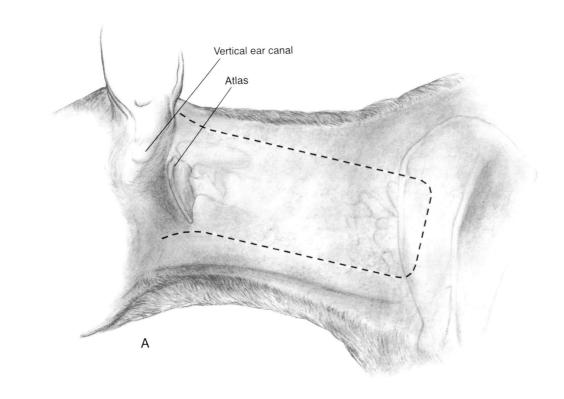

Vertical ear canal

Atlas

A

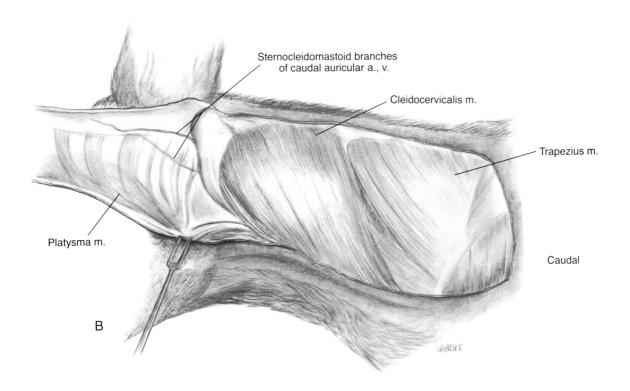

Sternocleidomastoid branches
of caudal auricular a., v.

Cleidocervicalis m.

Trapezius m.

Platysma m.

Caudal

B

Approach to the Omocervical Artery

INDICATIONS

Axial pattern flap for wound reconstruction involving the pinna, the face, the shoulder, and the cervical and axillary areas.

DESCRIPTION OF THE PROCEDURE

A. The patient is positioned in lateral recumbency, and the forelimb is placed in a relaxed position perpendicular to the trunk. A caudal skin incision is made over the spine of the scapula in a dorsal direction. The cranial skin incision is made parallel to the caudal incision equal to the distance between the scapular spine and the cranial shoulder depression, which is the location of the omocervical artery and vein. The dorsal incision site varies according to the size of the flap needed, but it may be made anywhere from the dorsal midline to the contralateral shoulder joint. A ventral incision is made at the level of the scapulohumeral joint to create an island arterial flap for additional mobility.

B. The flap is elevated below portions of the sphincter colli superficialis muscle and the subcutaneous tissue beginning dorsally. Care is taken to avoid trauma to the omocervical artery and vein arising from the cranial shoulder depression.

CLOSURE

The donor site is closed by apposition of the subcutaneous tissue with absorbable suture in an interrupted or continuous pattern. The skin is closed with nonabsorbable suture in a simple interrupted pattern. A soft rubber drain is placed in the wound, and the flap is sutured into the wound defect with nonabsorbable suture in a simple interrupted pattern. A subcutaneous closure is not performed on the flap to avoid compromise of vascular supply to the flap edges.

COMMENTS

A bridge incision is made between the donor bed and the wound site.

The flap described is the island arterial flap. A standard peninsula flap is constructed without making the fourth ventral incision.

Based on a procedure of Pavletic MM: Canine axial pattern flaps, using the omocervical, thoracodorsal, and deep circumflex iliac direct cutaneous arteries. Am J Vet Res 42:391, 1981.

Plate 110

Approach to the Omocervical Artery

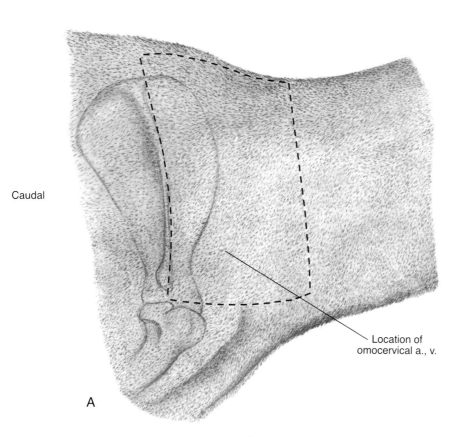

Caudal

Location of
omocervical a., v.

A

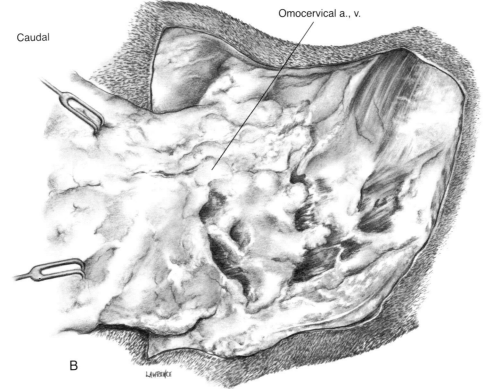

Caudal

Omocervical a., v.

B

LAWRENCE

Approach to the Thoracodorsal Artery

INDICATIONS

Axial pattern flap for wound reconstruction involving the thorax, the shoulder, the forelimb, and the axillary areas.

DESCRIPTION OF THE PROCEDURE

A. The patient is positioned in lateral recumbency, with the forelimb in relaxed extension. A cranial skin incision is made over the spine of the scapula in a dorsal direction. The caudal skin incision is made parallel to the cranial incision equal to the distance between the scapular spine and the caudal scapular edge. The dorsal incision site varies according to the size of the flap needed, but it may be made on the dorsal midline in most cases.

B. The flap is elevated below the level of the cutaneous trunci muscle and the subcutaneous tissue beginning dorsally. The thoracodorsal artery and vein arise from the caudal shoulder depression at a level parallel to the acromion. Care is taken to avoid these vessels, which are surrounded by abundant subcutaneous fat.

CLOSURE

The donor site is closed by apposition of the subcutaneous tissue with absorbable suture in a continuous or interrupted pattern. The skin is closed with nonabsorbable suture in a simple interrupted pattern. A soft rubber drain is placed in the wound, and the flap is sutured into the wound defect with nonabsorbable suture in a simple interrupted pattern. A subcutaneous closure is not performed on the flap to avoid possible compromise of vascular supply to the flap edges.

COMMENTS

A bridge incision is made between the donor bed and the wound site.

The flap described is the standard peninsula configuration. The flap may be modified to an L-shaped ("hockey stick") configuration with a right angle extension enabling the surgeon to cover irregular or wider defects. An island flap may be created by incision of the fourth side of the flap, which allows additional mobility.

Based on a procedure of Pavletic MM: Canine axial pattern flaps, using the omocervical, thoracodorsal, and deep circumflex iliac direct cutaneous arteries. Am J Vet Res 42:391, 1981.

Plate 111
Approach to the Thoracodorsal Artery

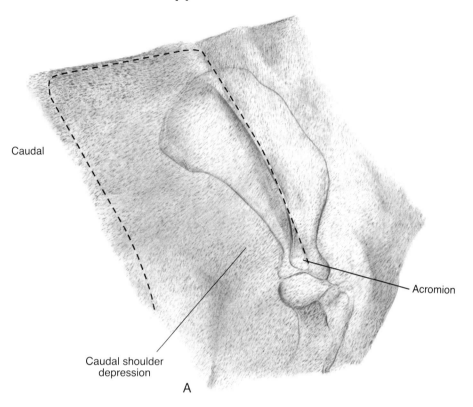

Caudal

Acromion

Caudal shoulder
depression

A

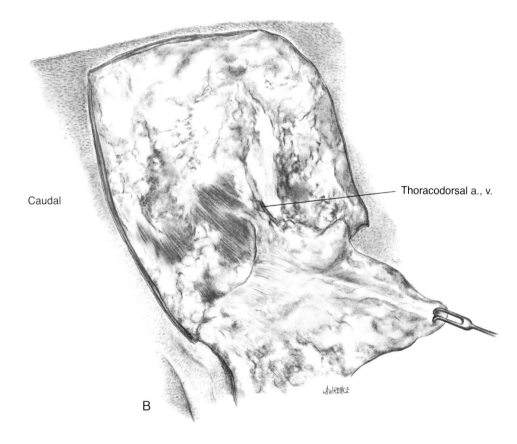

Caudal

Thoracodorsal a., v.

LAWRENCE

B

Approach to the Superficial Brachial Artery

INDICATIONS

Axial pattern flap for wound reconstruction involving the antebrachium and the elbow.

DESCRIPTION OF THE PROCEDURE

A. The patient is positioned in lateral recumbency, with the forelimb elevated and positioned perpendicular to the long axis of the body. The skin flap base is 5 to 6 cm wide and is centered over the flexor surface of the elbow. Craniomedial and caudolateral skin incisions are made parallel to the shaft of the humerus, extending proximally to the greater tubercle. The apex of the flap is narrower than the base to facilitate donor site wound closure.

B. The proximal skin incisions are joined, and the flap is elevated from proximal to distal with dissecting scissors. Care is taken to avoid the superficial brachial artery and vein, which enter the flap distally on the medial aspect of the elbow.

CLOSURE

The donor site is closed by apposition of the subcutaneous tissue with absorbable suture in a continuous or interrupted pattern. The skin is closed with nonabsorbable suture in a simple interrupted pattern. A soft rubber drain is placed in the wound, and the flap is sutured into the wound defect with nonabsorbable suture in a simple interrupted pattern. A subcutaneous closure is not performed on the flap to avoid possible compromise of vascular supply to the flap edges.

COMMENTS

A bridge incision is made between the donor bed and the wound site.

Survival of 95% to 100% of the length of the flap is expected.

The apex of the flap may be widened to improve wound coverage; however, additional undermining of skin edges will be necessary to close the donor site.

Based on a procedure of Shields-Henney LH, and Pavletic MM: Axial pattern flap based on the superficial brachial artery in the dog. Vet Surg 17:311, 1988.

Plate 112
Approach to the Superficial Brachial Artery

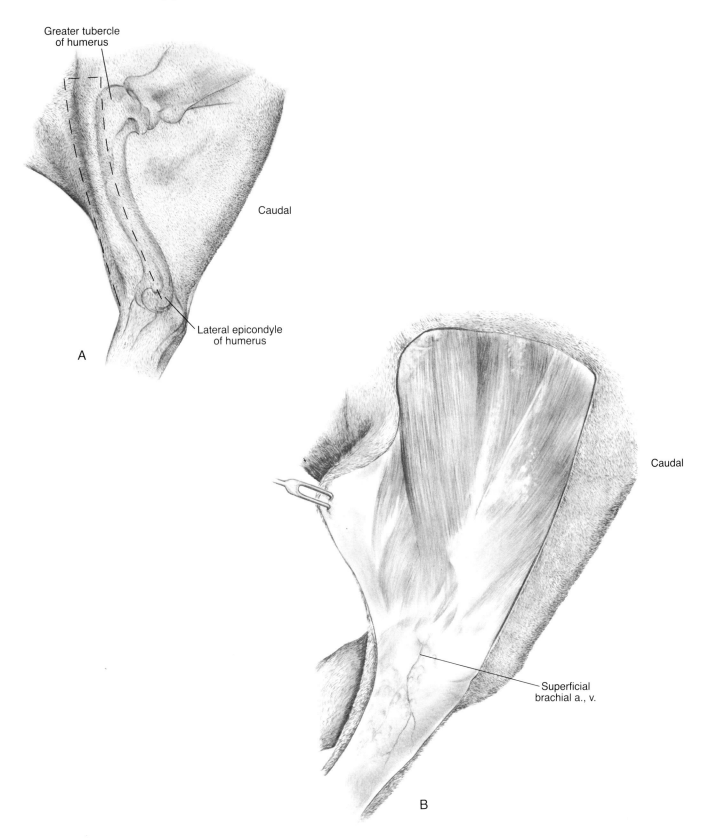

Greater tubercle
of humerus

Caudal

Lateral epicondyle
of humerus

A

Caudal

Superficial
brachial a., v.

B

Approach to the Caudal Superficial Epigastric Artery

INDICATIONS

Axial pattern flap for wound reconstruction involving the caudolateral flank, the medial thigh, and the stifle, inguinal, and perineal areas.

DESCRIPTION OF THE PROCEDURE

A. The patient is positioned in dorsal recumbency, and the hindlimbs are secured to the operating table in a frog-leg position. A midline abdominal skin incision is made beginning 3 to 4 cm caudal to the last mammary teat, continuing cranially to between mammary glands 2 and 3. The incision is then continued laterally and caudally at an equal distance lateral to the mammary teats parallel to the midline incision.

B. The surgeon undermines the flap from cranial to caudal with dissecting scissors, staying close to the external fascia of the rectus abdominis muscle and the aponeurosis of the external abdominal oblique muscle. Care is taken to avoid the caudal superficial epigastric artery and vein, which enter the flap caudally and are surrounded by inguinal fat.

CLOSURE

The donor site is closed by apposition of the subcutaneous tissue with absorbable suture in a continuous or interrupted pattern. The skin is closed with nonabsorbable suture in a simple interrupted pattern. A soft rubber drain is placed in the wound, and the flap is sutured into the wound defect with nonabsorbable suture in a simple interrupted pattern. A subcutaneous closure is not performed on the flap to avoid possible compromise of vascular supply to the flap edges.

COMMENTS

A bridge incision is made between the donor bed and the wound site.

In male dogs, the medial skin incision is made along the dorsal base of the preputial sheath and continued cranially along the abdominal midline.

The cranial aspect of the incision may be extended to between mammary glands 1 and 2 if desired. The medial and lateral flap incisions may be connected caudal to the last mammary gland to create an island arterial flap, which allows additional mobility.

Based on a procedure of Pavletic MM: Caudal superficial epigastric arterial pedicle grafts in the dog. Vet Surg 9:103, 1980.

Plate 113

Approach to the Caudal Superficial Epigastric Artery

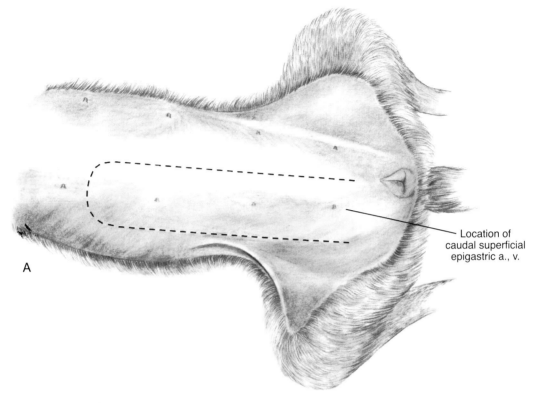

Location of
caudal superficial
epigastric a., v.

A

Caudal

Caudal superficial
epigastric a., v.

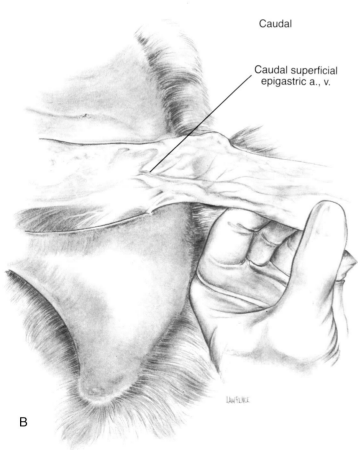

B

Approach to the Deep Circumflex Iliac Artery

INDICATIONS

Axial pattern flap for wound reconstruction involving the caudal thorax, the lateral abdominal wall, the flank, the lateral and medial thigh, and the greater trochanter area.

DESCRIPTION OF THE PROCEDURE

A. The patient is positioned in lateral recumbency, and the hindlimb is placed in relaxed extension perpendicular to the trunk. The caudal skin incision is made in a dorsoventral direction midway between the greater trochanter and the cranial aspect of the wing of the ilium. The cranial skin incision is made parallel to the caudal one, equal to the distance between the cranial iliac border and the caudal incision. The dorsal incision is made on the midline, or the flap may extend to the dorsal aspect of the contralateral flank skin fold. An island arterial flap is created by making a ventral incision just dorsal to the ipsilateral flank skin fold.

B. The flap is elevated below the cutaneous trunci muscle and the subcutaneous tissue beginning at the distal aspect. Care is taken to avoid the deep circumflex iliac vessels, which arise from a point just cranioventral to the wing of the ilium.

CLOSURE

The donor site is closed by apposition of the subcutaneous tissue with absorbable suture in a continuous or interrupted pattern. The skin is closed with nonabsorbable suture in a simple interrupted pattern. A soft rubber drain is placed in the wound, and the flap is sutured into the wound defect with nonabsorbable suture in a simple interrupted pattern. A subcutaneous closure is not performed on the flap to avoid possible compromise of vascular supply to the flap edges.

COMMENTS

A bridge incision is made between the donor bed and the wound site.

The flap described is the island arterial flap. A peninsula flap is constructed without making the ventral incision. An L-shaped ("hockey stick") incision may be made, depending on the location of the defect.

The deep circumflex iliac artery has both dorsal and ventral branches. The flap described is based on the dorsal arterial branch. The ventral branch also may be used for wound reconstruction, but clinical use is limited by its flank location.

Based on a procedure of Pavletic MM: Canine axial pattern flaps, using the omocervical, thoracodorsal, and deep circumflex iliac direct cutaneous arteries. Am J Vet Res 42:391, 1981.

Plate 114

Approach to the Deep Circumflex Iliac Artery

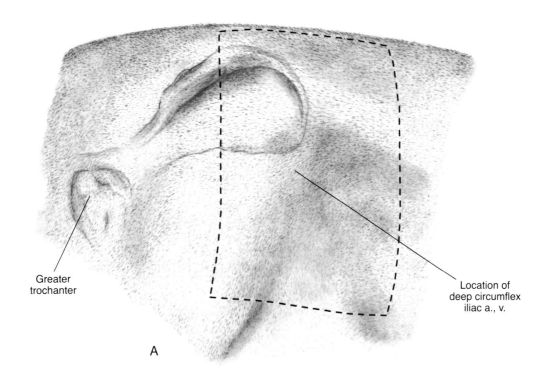

Greater
trochanter

Location of
deep circumflex
iliac a., v.

A

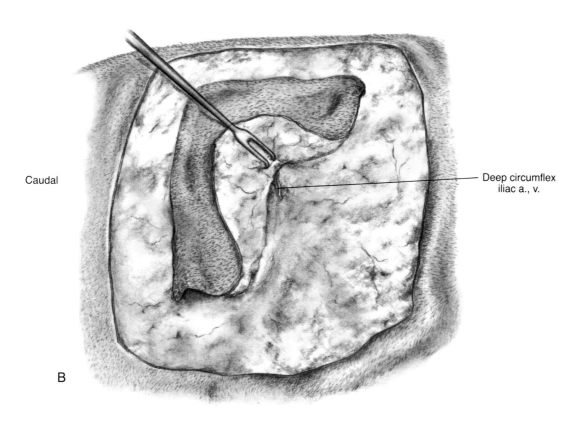

Caudal

Deep circumflex
iliac a., v.

B

Approach to the Medial Genicular Artery

INDICATIONS

Axial pattern flap for wound reconstruction involving the lateral and medial aspects of the hindlimb from the stifle to the tarsocrural joint.

DESCRIPTION OF THE PROCEDURE

A. The patient is positioned in lateral recumbency, with the hindlimb perpendicular to the long axis of the body. A skin incision is made beginning 2 cm proximal to the patella, extending proximally parallel to the shaft of the femur. A parallel incision is made beginning 1 to 1.5 cm distal to the tibial tuberosity, extending proximally to the level of the greater trochanter. The cranial and caudal skin incisions are joined by a proximal skin incision over the base of the greater trochanter.

B. The surgeon undermines the skin flap from proximal to distal with dissection scissors, staying close to the fascia lata and the biceps femoris muscle fascia. Care is taken to avoid the medial genicular artery, which enters the flap distally on the craniomedial aspect of the stifle.

CLOSURE

The donor site is closed by apposition of the subcutaneous tissue with absorbable suture in a continuous or interrupted pattern. The skin is closed with nonabsorbable suture in a simple interrupted pattern. A soft rubber drain is placed in the wound, and the flap is sutured into the wound defect with nonabsorbable suture in a simple interrupted pattern. A subcutaneous closure is not performed on the flap to avoid possible compromise of vascular supply to the flap edges.

COMMENTS

A bridge incision is made to connect the donor bed and the wound site.

Incisional dehiscence may occur at the level of the greater trochanter or at the T-shaped area where the donor and recipient sites meet. Inserting tension sutures, decreasing flap length, and placing the animal on a padded surface may minimize dehiscence.

Owing to variations in the number and the location of the genicular branches of the saphenous artery, necrosis may affect 10% to 30% of the length of the flaps.

Based on a procedure of Kostolich M, and Pavletic MM: Axial pattern flap based on the genicular branch of the saphenous artery in the dog. Vet Surg 16:217, 1987.

Plate 115
Approach to the Medial Genicular Artery

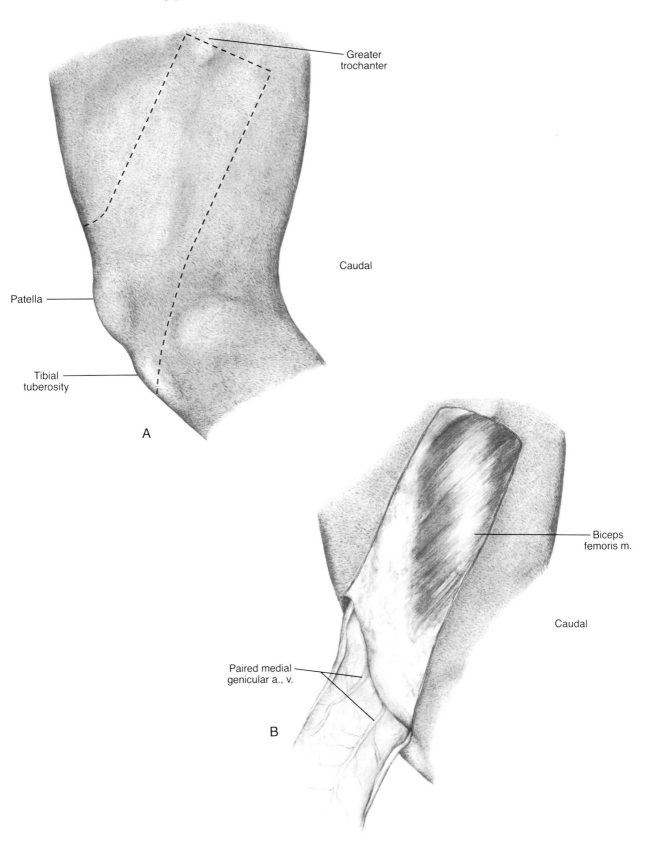

Greater
trochanter

Caudal

Patella

Tibial
tuberosity

A

Biceps
femoris m.

Caudal

Paired medial
genicular a., v.

B

Approach to the Lateral Caudal Artery

INDICATIONS

Axial pattern flap for wound reconstruction involving the caudodorsal trunk and perineal areas.

DESCRIPTION OF THE PROCEDURE

A. The patient is positioned in dorsal recumbency. A skin incision is made extending the full length of the tail on the dorsal midline. The flap is developed from the incision margins. The subcutaneous tissues are dissected from the deep caudal fascia, with care being taken to preserve the right and left lateral caudal arteries and veins.

B. The tail is amputated at the caudal 3rd or 4th vertebral interspace. The median caudal artery and dorsal lateral caudal arteries are ligated on the tail stump with absorbable suture.

CLOSURE

A soft rubber drain is placed in the wound, and the flap is sutured into the wound with nonabsorbable suture in a simple interrupted pattern. The base of the flap is utilized for tail stump closure with nonabsorbable suture in a simple interrupted pattern.

COMMENTS

Other reconstructive surgical techniques may be used for wounds in the caudodorsal area of the trunk to avoid tail amputation. Examples are the caudal superficial epigastric and the deep circumflex iliac axial pattern flaps, as illustrated in Approach to the Caudal Superficial Epigastric Artery and Approach to the Deep Circumflex Iliac Artery (see pp 366, 368). Local flaps also may be used.

A ventral midline skin incision allows flap development for reconstruction of perineal wounds.

Based on a procedure of Smith MM, Carrig CB, Waldron DR, and Trevor PB: Direct cutaneous arterial supply to the tail in dogs. Am J Vet Res 53:145, 1992.

Plate 116
Approach to the Lateral Caudal Artery

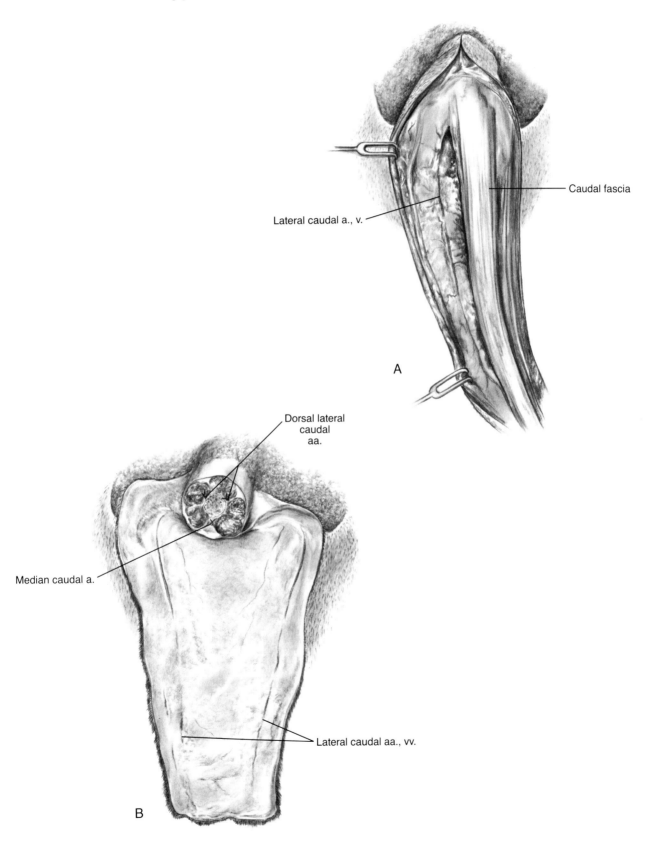

Caudal fascia

Lateral caudal a., v.

A

Dorsal lateral
caudal
aa.

Median caudal a.

Lateral caudal aa., vv.

B

Peripheral Lymphatic Surgery

- Approach to the Mandibular Lymph Node
- Approach to the Superficial Cervical Lymph Node
- Approach to the Superficial Inguinal Lymph Node
- Approach to the Popliteal Lymph Node

Approach to the Mandibular Lymph Node

INDICATIONS

Incisional or excisional biopsy of the mandibular lymph node to diagnose and/or stage neoplastic and inflammatory disease.

DESCRIPTION OF THE PROCEDURE

A. The patient is positioned in lateral recumbency. A skin incision is made beginning caudally at the bifurcation of the jugular vein and continuing cranially to the angle of the mandible.

Plate 117
Approach to the Mandibular Lymph Node

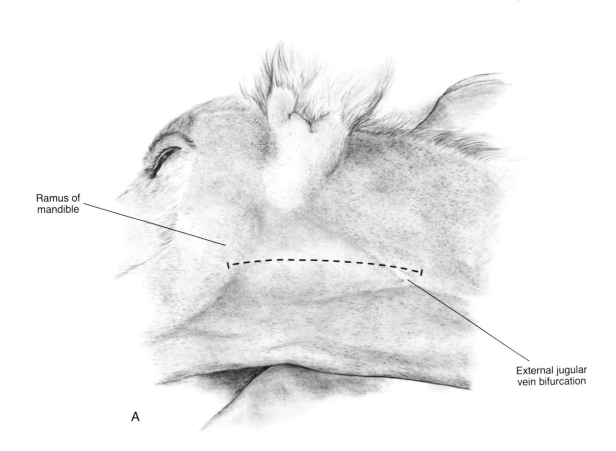

Ramus of
mandible

External jugular
vein bifurcation

A

Approach to the Mandibular Lymph Node *continued*

DESCRIPTION OF THE PROCEDURE *continued*

B. The incision is carried through the thin platysma muscle, and the mandibular salivary gland is identified between the maxillary and linguofacial veins. The largest of the mandibular lymph nodes in the normal dog is located cranial and ventral to the mandibular salivary gland.

C. The mandibular lymph node chain continues ventrally and caudally. The node or nodes are freed from surrounding tissue by a combination of sharp and blunt dissection. Blood vessels supplying the lymph node are ligated or cauterized.

CLOSURE

The subcutaneous tissue is closed with synthetic absorbable suture in a continuous pattern, and the skin is closed with nonabsorbable suture in a simple interrupted pattern.

COMMENTS

The mandibular lymph node chain consists variably of two to five nodes.

The mandibular salivary gland should *not* be mistaken for a lymph node. The salivary gland is larger, lobulated, and tan.

Plate 117

Approach to the Mandibular Lymph Node *continued*

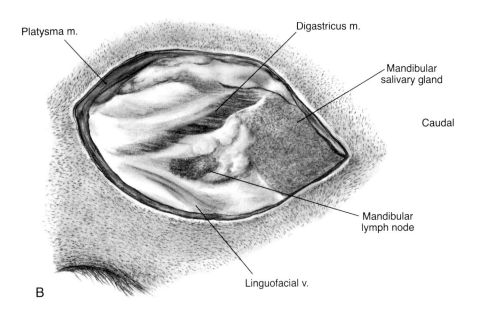

Platysma m.

Digastricus m.

Mandibular
salivary gland

Caudal

Mandibular
lymph node

Linguofacial v.

B

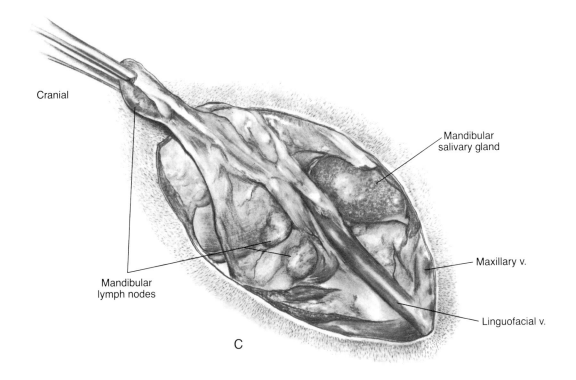

Cranial

Mandibular
salivary gland

Mandibular
lymph nodes

Maxillary v.

Linguofacial v.

C

Approach to the Superficial Cervical Lymph Node

INDICATIONS

Incisional or excisional biopsy of the superficial cervical lymph node to diagnose and/or stage neoplastic and inflammatory disease.

DESCRIPTION OF THE PROCEDURE

A. The patient is positioned in lateral recumbency. A 5- 6-cm skin incision is made just cranial to the scapula and dorsal to the greater tubercle of the humerus at the level of the acromion.

B. The platysma muscle and the subcutaneous tissue are incised, and the omotransversarius and brachiocephalicus muscles are identified.

Plate 118
Approach to the Superficial Cervical Lymph Node

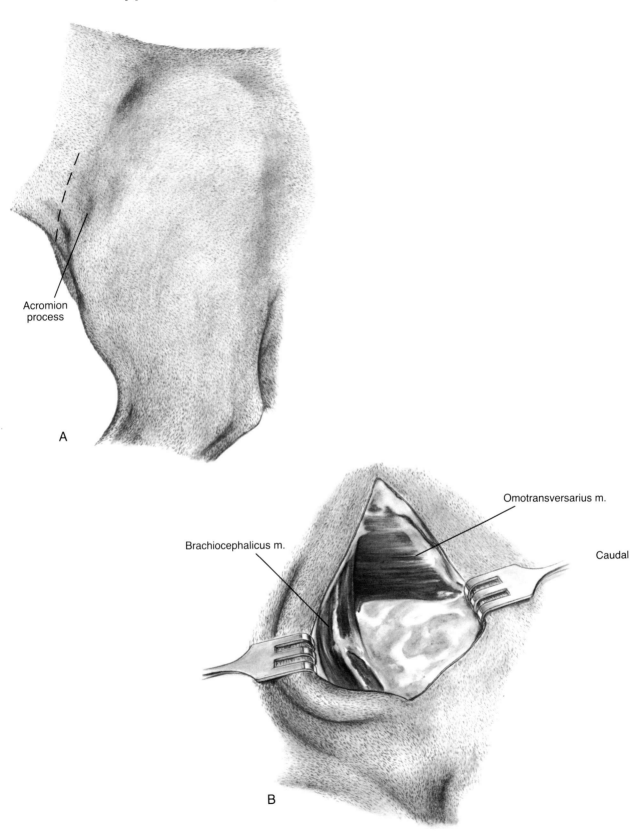

Acromion
process

A

Brachiocephalicus m.

Omotransversarius m.

Caudal

B

Approach to the Superficial Cervical Lymph Node *continued*

DESCRIPTION OF THE PROCEDURE *continued*

C. The node normally lies in fat between the two muscles. A combination of sharp and blunt dissection is used to free the lymph node from its loose attachments. The blood vessels supplying the node are ligated or cauterized.

CLOSURE

The subcutaneous tissues are apposed with absorbable suture in a continuous or interrupted pattern. The skin is closed with nonabsorbable suture in a simple interrupted pattern. If the node is greatly enlarged, dead space is closed with several absorbable sutures in an interrupted pattern.

Plate 118

Approach to the Superficial Cervical Lymph Node *continued*

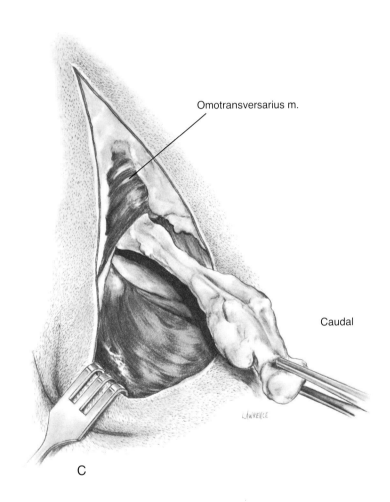

C

Approach to the Superficial Inguinal Lymph Node

INDICATIONS

Incisional or excisional biopsy of the superficial inguinal lymph node to diagnose and/ or stage neoplastic and inflammatory disease.

DESCRIPTION OF THE PROCEDURE

A. The patient is positioned in dorsal recumbency, with the rear limbs in a frog-leg position. A skin incision is made over the inguinal ring lateral to the fifth teat in the female and lateral to the prepuce in the male.

B. The subcutaneous tissue is incised to expose the vaginal process, the abundant fat of the inguinal region, and the abdominal fascia. Care is taken during lymph node excision or biopsy to avoid the external pudendal and caudal superficial epigastric arteries and veins. Blood vessels supplying the lymph node are ligated if excision is performed.

CLOSURE

The subcutaneous tissue is closed with absorbable suture in a continuous or interrupted pattern. The skin is closed with nonabsorbable suture in an interrupted pattern.

COMMENTS

There may be one or two superficial inguinal lymph nodes.

If the node is markedly enlarged, the skin incision may be made directly over the palpated node.

Plate 119

Approach to the Superficial Inguinal Lymph Node

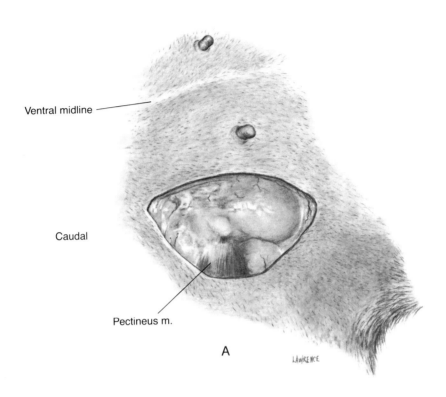

Ventral midline

Caudal

Pectineus m.

A

LAWRENCE

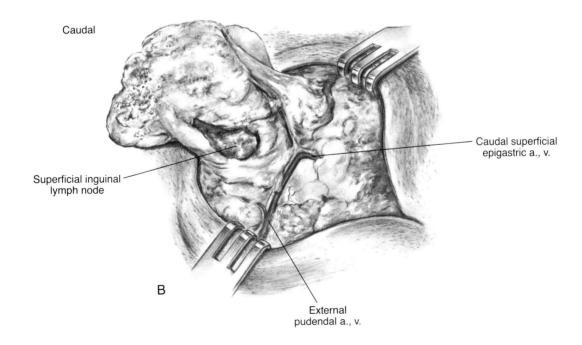

Caudal

Superficial inguinal
lymph node

Caudal superficial
epigastric a., v.

External
pudendal a., v.

B

Approach to the Popliteal Lymph Node

INDICATIONS

Incisional or excisional biopsy of the popliteal lymph node to diagnose and/or stage neoplastic and inflammatory disease.

DESCRIPTION OF THE PROCEDURE

A. The patient is positioned in lateral recumbency, with the affected limb placed uppermost in an elevated position. A skin incision is made directly over the lymph node, which is located in the popliteal space caudal to the stifle joint.

B. The node lies in fat and is located between the borders of the biceps femoris and semitendinosus muscles. If excision of the node is elected, a combination of sharp and blunt dissection is used to free the lymph node from its loose attachments. The blood vessels supplying the node are ligated or cauterized.

CLOSURE

The subcutaneous tissues are closed with absorbable suture in a continuous or interrupted pattern. The skin is closed with nonabsorbable suture in a simple interrupted pattern.

COMMENTS

Rear limb edema occasionally results from lymph node excision. The edema is nonpathologic and resolves slowly with ambulation and development of collateral lymphatic drainage.

Plate 120
Approach to the Popliteal Lymph Node

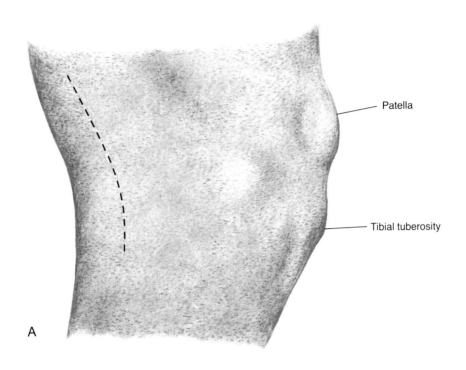

Patella

Tibial tuberosity

A

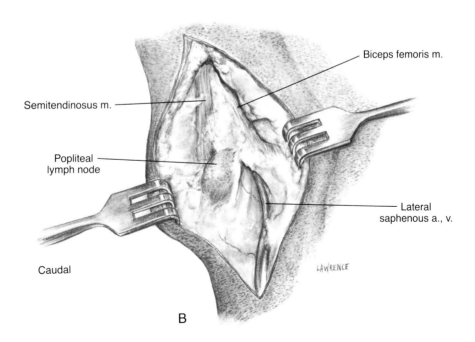

Semitendinosus m.

Popliteal
lymph node

Caudal

Biceps femoris m.

Lateral
saphenous a., v.

LAWRENCE

B

Index

Note: Page numbers in *italics* refer to illustrations.

Abdomen, approach to, by caudoventral midline celiotomy,
    in female dog, 172, *173*
    in male dog, 174, *175*, 176, *177*
  by cranioventral midline celiotomy, 166, *167*, 168, *169*
  by cranioventral-paracostal celiotomy, 170, *171*
  by paralumbar celiotomy, 178, *179*, 180, *181*
Abdominal oblique muscle(s), external, in approach to right
      caudal thorax, by ninth intercostal space
      thoracotomy, *135*
    in approach to right thorax, by fifth intercostal space
      thoracotomy, *131, 133*
  fibers of, in approach to abdomen, by cranioventral mid-
      line celiotomy, *169*
        by paralumbar celiotomy, *179, 181*
    in approach to inguinal ring, *301*
Abdominal surgery, 164–253
Abdominal wall, lateral, wound reconstruction on, 368, *369*
Acoustic meatus, external, in approach to ear canal, *3*
Acromial process, in approach to thoracodorsal artery, *363*
Adductor muscle, in approach to hindlimb for amputation,
    325, 327
Adenoma, of thyroid, *109*
Adrenal gland(s), approach to, 224–230, *225–231*
Adrenalectomy, by paralumbar celiotomy, 178, *179*, 180, *181*
Alimentation, parenteral, approach for, 338, *339*
Alveolar nerve, inferior, in approach to hemimandible, *71*
Amputation, of dewclaw, 330, *331*
  of forelimb, 318–322, *319–323*
  of forequarter, 310–316, *311–317*
  of hindlimb, 324, *325*, 326, *327*
  of tail, 328, *329*
  of third phalanx, feline, 332, *333*
Anal sac(s), approach to, canine, 292, *293*
Anal sphincter muscle(s), in approach to anal sacs, canine,
    293
  in approach to lateral perineum, 303, *305*
  in approach to pelvic canal, *205*
  in approach to rectum, *205*
Angiography, approach for, 338, *339*
  cranial, approach to, 336, *337*
  of hindlimb, approach to, 334, *335*
Antebrachium, wound reconstruction of, 364, *365*
Aorta, bifurcation with caudal vena cava, in approach to
      medial iliac lymph nodes, *251*
  in approach to caudal thorax, by transdiaphragmatic tho-
      racotomy, *143*
  in intrathoracic approach to left heart base, *151*

Aorta *(Continued)*
  in intrathoracic approach to right caudal esophagus, *163*
  in intrathoracic approach to thoracic duct, *163*
Artery(ies). See also specific arteries, e.g., *Femoral artery.*
  approach to, 334, *335*
Arytenoid cartilage, in approach to larynx, *35*
  lateralization of, 44, *45*, 46, *47*
  muscular process of, suture in, *47*
Arytenoidectomy, partial, approach for, 34, *35*
Atlas, in approach to caudal auricular artery, *359*
Auricle, right, approach to, intrathoracic, 154, *155*, 156, *157*
Auricular artery, caudal, approach to, 358, *359*
Auricular vein, caudal, in approach to parotid salivary
      gland, *89*
    sternocleidomastoid branch of, *359*
Axial pattern flap(s), in approach to caudal auricular artery,
    358, *359*
  in approach to caudal superficial epigastric artery, 366,
    367
  in approach to deep circumflex iliac artery, 368, *369*
  in approach to lateral caudal artery, 372, *373*
  in approach to medial genicular artery, 370, *371*
  in approach to omocervical artery, 360, *361*
  in approach to superficial brachial artery, 364, *365*
  in approach to thoracodorsal artery, 362, *363*
Axillary artery, in approach to forequarter for amputation,
    317
Axillary lymph node(s), in approach to forequarter for
      amputation, *317*
Axillary nerve, in approach to forelimb for amputation, *321*
Axillary vein, in approach to forequarter for amputation,
    317
Azygos vein, in approach to mediastinal lymph nodes, *153*
  in approach to right cranial esophagus, *153*
  in approach to trachea, *153*
  in intrathoracic approach to hilus of right lung, *161*
  in intrathoracic approach to tracheal bifurcation, *159*
  in intrathoracic approach to tracheobronchial lymph
      nodes, *159*

Basihyoid bone, in approach to ventral larynx, *43*
Basipharyngeal canal, in approach to nasal turbinates,
    canine, *25*
Biceps brachii muscle, in approach to forelimb for
    amputation, *323*

389